ADOLESCENT VULNERABILITIES AND OPPORTUNITIES

This book explores the central importance of adolescents' own activities in their development. This focus harkens back to Jean Piaget's genetic epistemology and provides a theoretically coherent vision of what makes adolescence a distinctive period of development, with unique opportunities and vulnerabilities. An interdisciplinary and international group of contributors explore how adolescents integrate neurological, cognitive, personal, interpersonal, and social systems aspects of development into more organized systems.

Eric Amsel is University Distinguished Professor and Chair of the Psychology Department at Weber State University. He has published three other books: *The Development of Scientific Thinking Skills* (1998, with Deanna Kuhn and Michael O'Loughlin); *Change and Development: Issues of Theory, Method and Application* (1998, with K. Ann Renninger); and *Language, Literacy, and Cognitive Development: The Development and Consequences of Symbolic Communication* (2002, with James P. Byrnes). He has published more than twenty journal articles in such journals as *Child Development, Cognition, Cognitive Development, Developmental Psychology, Journal of Research in Adolescence,* and *New Ideas in Psychology.* Amsel is Associate Editor of *New Ideas in Psychology.* He also serves as a Board Member and is a past Vice President of the Jean Piaget Society.

Judith Smetana has published six other books: *Adolescents, Families, and Social Development: How Adolescents Construct Their Worlds* (2011); *Social Development, Social Inequalities, and Social Justice* (2008, with Elliot Turiel and Cecilia Wainryb); *New Directions for Child Development: Changing Boundaries of Parental Authority during Adolescence* (2005); *Handbook of Moral Development* (2005, with Melanie Killen); *Parental Beliefs: Causes and Consequences for Development* (1994); and *Concepts of Self and Morality: Women's Reasoning about Abortion* (1982). She has published more than seventy articles in such journals as *Child Development, Developmental Psychology, Human Development, Journal of Adolescence, Journal of Research in Adolescence, Journal of Family Psychology,* and *Social Development.* Smetana has served as Associate Editor of *Child Development* and is on the editorial board of *Child Development, Developmental Psychology, Human Development, Journal of Adolescent Research, Parenting: Science and Practice,* and *Social Development.*

INTERDISCIPLINARY PERSPECTIVES ON KNOWLEDGE AND DEVELOPMENT: THE JEAN PIAGET SYMPOSIUM SERIES

Series Editor: Nancy Budwig, *Clark University*

Current titles: Published by Cambridge University Press

Adolescent Vulnerabilities and Opportunities: Developmental and Constructivist Perspectives, edited by Eric Amsel and Judith Smetana, 2011.

Prior Editors: Lynn S. Liben and Ellin Kofsky Scholnick

Published by Lawrence Erlbaum Associates/ Taylor and Francis/ Psychology Press

Art and Human Development, edited by Constance Milbrath and Cynthia Lightfoot, 2009.

Developmental Social Cognitive Neuroscience, edited by Philip David Zelazo, Michael Chandler, and Eveline Crone, 2009.

Social Life and Social Knowledge: Toward a Process Account of Development, edited by Ulrich Mueller, Jeremy I.M. Carpendale, Nancy Budwig, and Bryan Sokol, 2009.

Social Development, Social Inequalities, and Social Justice, edited by Cecilia Wainryb, Judith G. Smetana, and Elliot Turiel, 2007.

Developmental Perspectives on Embodiment and Consciousness, edited by Willis Overton, Ulrich Mueller, and Judith Newman, 2007.

Play and Development: Evolutionary, Sociocultural, and Functional Perspectives, edited by Artin Goncu and Suzanne Gaskins, 2007.

Biology and Knowledge Revisited: From Neurogenesis to Psychogenesis, edited by Sue Taylor Parker, Jonas Langer, and Constance Milbrath, 2004.

Changing Conceptions of Psychological Life, edited by Cynthia Lightfoot, Michael Chandler, and Chris Lalonde, 2004.

Language, Literacy, and Cognitive Development, edited by Eric Amsel and James P. Byrnes, 2003.

Reductionism and the Development of Knowledge, edited by Terrance Brown and Leslie Smith, 2002.

Culture, Thought, and Development, edited by Larry Nucci, Geoffrey B. Saxe, and Elliot Turiel, 2000.

(*continued after the Index*)

Adolescent Vulnerabilities and Opportunities

DEVELOPMENTAL AND CONSTRUCTIVIST PERSPECTIVES

Edited by

Eric Amsel

Weber State University

Judith Smetana

University of Rochester

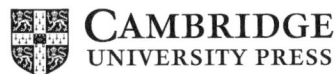

CAMBRIDGE
UNIVERSITY PRESS

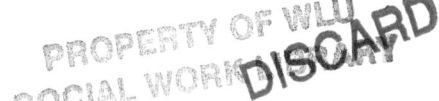

CAMBRIDGE UNIVERSITY PRESS
Cambridge, New York, Melbourne, Madrid, Cape Town,
Singapore, São Paulo, Delhi, Tokyo, Mexico City

Cambridge University Press
32 Avenue of the Americas, New York, NY 10013-2473, USA

www.cambridge.org
Information on this title: www.cambridge.org/9780521768467

© Cambridge University Press 2011

First published 2011

Printed in the United States of America

A catalog record for this publication is available from the British Library.

Library of Congress Cataloging in Publication data
Adolescent vulnerabilities and opportunities: developmental and constructivist
perspectives / [edited by] Eric Amsel, Judith Smetana.
p.   cm.
Includes bibliographical references and index.
ISBN 978-0-521-76846-7 (hbk.)
1. Adolescent psychology.   2. Adolescence.   3. Constructivism (Psychology)
I. Amsel, Eric.   II. Smetana, Judith G., 1951–   III. Title.
BF724.A278   2011
155.5–dc22   2011008037

ISBN 978-0-521-76846-7 Hardback

Contents

Figures and Tables

FIGURES

TABLES

Series Editor's Preface

In 1970, Jean Piaget participated in a workshop that instigated vigorous discussion in higher education circles about the importance of traversing the boundaries across the disciplines. The workshop, entitled "L'interdiscip linarité – Problèmes d'enseignement et de recherche dans les universities," was held in Nice, France, in September 1970 and the proceedings were published in 1972 as a monograph entitled *Interdisciplinarity: Problems of Teaching and Research in Universities* (Paris: Organization for Economic Cooperation and Development). This workshop and the book that resulted from it set the stage for ongoing debates about how best to view work going on at the intersection of disciplinary boundaries. Piaget's remarks made clear that new conceptual frameworks were needed, frameworks that underscored the importance of augmenting disciplinary knowledge in order to address the enduring challenges of our times. Whether to do so from multi-, trans-, or interdisciplinary bases and what precisely each of these constructs adds to disciplinary discussions has been hotly debated for the ensuing four decades. What Piaget was wrestling with in 1970 and many others have been pursuing since then are two enduring issues: the complexity of knowledge and the importance of viewing knowledge construction as a process embedded in real time. Piaget understood early on what has become more obvious now, namely the importance of going beyond disciplinary limitations both theoretically and methodologically. This insight has shaped modern thinking on knowledge and development in significant ways.

Around the same time that Piaget spoke at the OECD workshop, a new society was formed. In 1970, the Jean Piaget Society was founded. It has since provided an internationally recognized forum for inquiry about and advances of significant problems in the developmental sciences. The Society has had a long-standing commitment to developmental perspectives and has been deeply concerned with theories and conceptualizations of development and the ways developmental perspectives connect to and influence research. Since renamed The Jean Piaget Society for Knowledge and Development, the Society organizes and sponsors a book series, an annual meeting of plenary addresses and scholarly presentations, a scholarly journal (*Cognitive Development*), and a Web site (http://www.piaget. org). Across venues, participating scholars come from a range of disciplines, including departments of psychology, anthropology, linguistics, sociology, biology, philosophy, and education.

The Society has had a long-standing dedication to the publication of a book series that addresses core problems in the developmental sciences. For more than thirty years, Lawrence Erlbaum Press (currently Psychology Press/ Taylor and Francis) published the series, carefully edited for its first decade by Lynn S. Liben and then by Ellin Kofsky Scholnick. Each of the volumes in the Jean Piaget Symposium series engages well-recognized scholars on a set of themes that bring together divergent disciplinary perspectives. The series, which has included nearly forty published volumes, has dealt with topics such as human understanding, developmental psychopathology, concept formation, and relations between learning and development.

In a time when there appears to be a proliferation of edited volumes, one can ask what makes this series thrive. The high regard for these volumes has been due to the careful way interdisciplinary thinking has shed light on enduring issues with which scholars interested in human development are grappling. To a large measure the rigorous system of cultivation and review plays a significant role in arriving at cutting-edge thinking that goes beyond juxtaposition of new ideas. Careful attention is given to taking a theme at the center of developmental science (e.g., epigenesis of mind; culture, thought, and development; social development and social justice; developmental social cognitive neuroscience) and weaving scholarship from neighboring disciplines into discussions in ways that hold the potential to significantly shape ongoing scientific discourse.

Each of the JPS series volumes emanates from the Society's themed annual meeting that includes plenary addresses and invited symposia, a meeting structure that itself is the outcome of a long and rigorous academic review process. Typically, several revisions are made in the proposal before it obtains approval from the full Board of Directors. The annual meeting organizers also serve as editors of the volume. To supplement chapters by the five or six plenary speakers, the volume editors typically invite other contributors to the volume. The editors also inform contributors about the requirements with regard to the volume's theme and scope. Finally, the editors engage in a thorough evaluation of each contribution, providing extensive feedback and soliciting revisions until they are of the required quality. This process ensures that extraordinary scholars will contribute to the volumes. In summary, we believe the book series has provided a distinctive intellectual contribution to the study of knowledge and development by focusing on developmental inquiry from an interdisciplinary perspective. Further information about the series can be found at: http://www.piaget .org/Series/series.html.

The inaugural volume of our new book series Interdisciplinary Perspectives on Knowledge and Development: The Jean Piaget Symposium series with Cambridge University Press exemplifies the strong inter-disciplinary approach that has been central to all of our prior volumes. Edited by Eric Amsel and Judith Smetana, *Adolescent Vulnerabilities and Opportunities: Developmental and Constructivist Perspectives* continues the Jean Piaget Society's tradition of providing a recognized forum for advancing inquiry about both enduring and emergent problems in the developmental sciences. This volume brings together neurological, cognitive, self-system, moral, and social perspectives on adolescents' active processes for coordinating capacities, skills, and understandings. Greater than the sum of its parts, each chapter contributes to the larger conceptual framework contributing to redefining our understanding about this intriguing time of development. As such, this inaugural volume represents the goals of the series splendidly and paves the way for further interdisciplinary scholarship at the frontiers of new knowledge about human development.

Nancy Budwig, Clark University, Worcester, MA
December 2010

Preface

It was a brief conversation between the two of us in Atlanta at the Society for Research in Child Development in 2005 that set the wheels rolling and resulted in this book. It was a time of mounting excitement over new and broad-based findings about adolescent development, including new findings on adolescent brain development, risk taking, identity development, peer and family relations, and contextual and cultural influences. These findings were seen as evidence of biological and socio-contextual factors on adolescent development and further proof that a constructivist framework for understanding adolescent development, once in its ascendancy, is now in decline.

As developmental psychologists, we never found the new findings particularly incompatible with a broadly constructivist framework, a point we reaffirmed in our discussions in Atlanta. We decided then and there that there was value in organizing a conference on adolescent development from a constructivist perspective to make sense of the new findings. Our goal was to reinvigorate the constructivist approach to adolescent development, which we saw as being unnecessarily dismissed as irrelevant to research and theory in adolescence.

As members of the Board (JS) and Executive Committee (EA) of the Jean Piaget Society, we brought our proposal for a symposium to the subsequent board meeting. The proposal was met with positive comments and suggestions about the invited speakers and symposia. We thank the JPS board members and society leadership at the time (President Nancy Budwig, past President Elliot Turiel, and President-Elect Geoff Saxe) for their help in putting together the intellectual content of the conference and sharpening its conceptual focus.

The conference was held in Quebec City in June 2008, as the Thirty-Eighth Annual Meeting of the Jean Piaget Society. The hard work of putting on the conference was ably handled by the 2008 JPS executive committee, composed of Connie Milbrath (VP Publicity), Chris Lalonde (VP Information Technology), Colette Daiute (Secretary), and Ashley Maynard (Treasurer). Also, we extend our thanks to the many scholars who adjudicated the submitted program to the conference.

Our gratitude goes to the local arrangement team in Quebec City, led by Teresa Blicharski and assisted by Helene Ziarko, Simon Larose, Shephan Desrochers, and Margurtute Lavallee, all of Laval University. Together with an army of their graduate and undergraduate student assistants, the local arrangements team ensured that the Quebec conference ran smoothly, down to the smallest detail.

We would also like to thank a number of institutions and people for their financial and professional support of the conference. The Social Science and Humanities Research Council of Canada generously supported the conference with a grant through the Aid to Research Workshops and Conferences in Canada program. Thanks are extended to Elsevier, Taylor and Francis, and the University of Laval for their financial support of the conference. Also, a special thanks to Lauren Greenfield, whose photographic work adorned the program and poster for the conference, and to Chris Lalonde and Bill Hallam for designing the program and poster. Finally, a thank you to Aubrey Jenkins and Jessamy Comer for their help preparing the volume and to Nancy Budwig from JPS and Amanda O'Connor from Cambridge for shepherding the manuscript through to publication.

There is an old saying from J. B. Priestley that goes: "Like its politicians and its wars, society has the teenagers it deserves." The purpose of this project was to better understand teenagers and help them negotiate their transition to adulthood. As editors we would like to thank our families (EA: Judi and the boys; JS: Ron and the boys) for not just tolerating but even supporting our preoccupation with this project and its goal.

December 16, 2010

Constructivist Processes in Adolescent Development

ERIC AMSEL

Weber State University

JUDITH G. SMETANA

University of Rochester

In John Godfrey Saxe's poem, *The Blind Men and the Elephant*, based on earlier Chinese and Indian fables, six blind men surround and feel some part of an elephant. Each of them thinks that his part reveals the true nature of the beast. Saxe makes clear that the lesson to be learned involves the dangers in generalizing knowledge claims that are limited in scope. This lesson translates well into research on adolescent development. Although adolescents are popularly seen as having an unpredictable and inexplicable nature, any good adolescence textbook documents a range of conflicting alternative images afforded by multiple theoretical perspectives in the field. Adolescents are presented as *apprentices* (who participate in forms of cultural activities), *architects* (who construct normative mental structures and processes), and *juveniles* (who accommodate to a long, slow biological maturation processes).[1]

Just as Saxe warns, each of the theoretical frameworks underlying these images highlights a particular set of factors or forces as central to understanding adolescence, which is in turn used to paint these generalized but conflicting pictures. For example, fifty or so years ago, adolescence was seen as time for acquiring morality, rationality, and an autonomous sense of self and identity (Erikson, 1968; Inhelder & Piaget, 1958; Kohlberg, 1969), a position articulately defended by Moshman (2005). The constructivist theoretical framework that underlies much of this work presents a view of adolescents as designing their own development by actively seeking to make sense of themselves and their physical and social worlds. These powerful ideas, and the image of adolescents as architects that they imply, gave rise to a research program defining the normative developmental trajectory in adolescence as a progression toward rationality, morality, and autonomy.

---

[1] Thanks to Cynthia Lightfoot for contributions to these metaphors.

Constructivists were not blind to the challenges that arise as adolescents confront the trials and tribulations of accommodating to puberty and adopting adult social roles. But the theoretical and empirical goal was to lay out the pathways leading toward developmental endpoints rather than charting the deviations, diversions, and detours in development.

However, by the 1970s, the impact of these "grand" theories of adolescent development slowly began to wane as research and theory were directed to the influence of biological (neurological and hormonal), individual (personality and emotional), and social (cultural and contextual) factors in explaining adolescent behavior (for a review, see Lerner & Steinberg, 2009). To Lerner and Steinberg (2009), this research reflected a shift in interest from normative developmental processes (what we alluded to as pathways to endpoints) to a focus on the diversity of biopsychosocial influences on adolescent behavior and on factors that promote particular culturally relevant outcomes. This attention to "deviations, diversions, and detours" in development was described in other adolescent frameworks as evidence of the diversity and plasticity of development in adolescence. It also was used to dispute the narrowly defined normative developmental pathways articulated by constructivists. All this took a toll on the viability of the image of adolescents as architects who construct various socio-cognitive competencies during their teen years. Instead, images of adolescents as *apprentices* and *juveniles* were refurbished after years of lying dormant.

In 2008, the Jean Piaget Society sponsored a conference specifically addressing the constructivist account of development in adolescence. Our goal was not to resurrect the old ideas about normative developmental pathways, as many of them have been revised since the 1950s. Rather, our goal was to reinvigorate interest in the core assumptions and features of the approach in a way that is responsive to the new biological, socio-relational, and sociocultural research. As will be more fully documented later, a major concern motivating the conference was that some of new work on the diversity and plasticity of adolescent development obscures what for constructivists is a core assumption about adolescence as a distinctive period of time in the life cycle, offering adolescents unique opportunities but also creating for them particular vulnerabilities.

As meeting organizers and now editors of this book, our goal was to further explore and reinvigorate a constructivist account of adolescent development. In this introductory chapter, we explore the attributes and processes of the constructivist approach to adolescent development that we think remain key in understanding adolescent behavior and development and the uniqueness of this life phase. We begin with an analysis of the constructivist approach in and critical features of genetic epistemology. Armed with some general constructivist principles of adolescent development, we address the constructivist vision of what makes adolescence a distinctive period of development, with unique opportunities and vulnerabilities. We then review the chapters of the book. Although not all of the contributors to this volume explicitly view their research as coming from a constructivist perspective, we believe that their work has much to offer such a view. We point out ways in which each of the chapters picks up on features of constructivism we lay out. We conclude with suggestions for future constructivist-oriented research on adolescent development.

CONSTRUCTIVISM AND GENETIC EPISTEMOLOGY

Constructivism holds that knowledge is derived from the physical or mental activity of the knower. The role of activity in the constructivist account of the acquisition of knowledge – for infants, adolescents, and octogenarians alike – implies that the nature of the knowledge acquired is intimately tied to the process of its acquisition. For example, if $2 + 1 = 3$ is acquired only as a contingent mathematical *fact*, its meaning and value for the knower is wholly dependent on the context in which it is learned and the source from whom it is learned. Presumably, it would matter whether the fact was learned in the classroom from a teacher as part of a formal lesson or as a casual comment from a sibling at home. The context, including the source's reasons for and trustworthiness in relaying the fact, may be part of what is known by the knower. In contrast, if $2 + 1 = 3$ is acquired as a necessary mathematical *truth*, its meaning and value for the knower lies in other mathematical procedures that can be performed on the expression (e.g., $3 - 2 = 1; 1 + 2 = 3; 3 - 1 = 2$) and organized into a coordinated set of procedures. The coordinated mathematical procedures, not the context, are then part of what is known by the knower. A number of central principles of Piaget's genetic epistemology emerge from this example of how knowers' activities affect their knowledge. We review some of these principles that, although not exhaustive, point out some key attributes of constructivism for adolescent development.

One genetic epistemological principle is that *the nature of the knower's activity is central to knowing*. In its most general sense, this is ingrained in Piaget's equilibration process, which holds that a person's knowledge *about* the world is altered (referred to as accommodation) just enough by new knowledge gathered *from* the world (referred to as assimilation) to permit the person to act effectively *in* the world. This effective action is a product of finding the right balance or equilibrium between accommodation and assimilation.

On the assimilation side, the level of activity in which the knower engages *constrains* what can be learned in the context. This refers to the Piagetian contention that learning is subordinate to development; cognitive development limits the forms and levels of activities that can be performed in a context. More advanced stages of cognitive (or social) development are associated with higher levels of activities, which promote more complete assimilation of knowledge.

On the accommodation side, activity level can be coordinated and abstracted into new forms of cognitive structures. According to genetic epistemology, coordinated activities may be projected onto a more abstract cognitive plane, thereby reorganizing cognitive structures. This is the Piagetian account of the emergence of advanced cognitive structures by the reflective abstraction of activities at one level onto a higher, more abstract level. For example, a knower's coordinated mathematical activities in learning that $3 - 1 = 2$ can be projected onto a higher plane by being transformed into logico-mathematical operations (e.g., reversibility and class inclusion), resulting in the transition to a more advanced stage of cognitive development.

By emphasizing individuals' activities in the acquisition of knowledge, Piaget's constructivism advocates an epistemological position that knowledge is neither innately preformed in the mind nor directly copied from the environment. But more than this, constructivism further advocates that individuals' activities simultaneously set *constraints* on learning in a particular context and *possibilities* of creating new cognitive structures. Of course, these constraints and possibilities shift and expand over time as new experiences are managed and challenges are overcome. But in setting constraints on learning and possibilities of development, a constructivist account of knowledge emphasizes the individual as an indispensible source of learning and development.

This point goes to the second important principle of Piaget's genetic epistemology, that individuals are not just active in knowing, but are *active agents in their own learning and development*. In constructivism, individuals are treated as self-organizing organisms (Reese & Overton, 1970), composed of structurally interrelated parts that form an integral whole. As a result, change and development originate in individuals' actions rather than directly from biological or environmental factors. Langer (1969, pp. 7–8) elegantly makes the point about the self-organizing nature of constructivist organisms:

The organism is a "self-organizing being": it has self-"*moving* power" and self- "formative power." Although the organism is not necessarily conscious of these powers, they permit it to generate or construct its own growth. It is as if the development of organisms represented a directedness towards ends immanent in their organization. This is possible because the most important characteristics of organic structures is that they have functions; that is, they are both agencies (means) for action and the end products (purposes) toward which action is directed.

In Piaget's constructivism, an active agent's *means* and *purposes* are intimately connected, resulting in local cognitive activities serving as a basis for transformed cognitive structures. They become more stable, powerful, and abstract, allowing for more effective future activities in the world. This leads us to a third principle, that *cognitive structures regulate behavior and do so in an increasingly effective manner over development*. As we have seen, cognitive structures function to regulate thought and behavior and are in turn a product of equilibration, improving its regulatory function. This improvement lies in cognitive structures supporting forms of activities, which are better at dealing with negative feedback once it occurs and are more effective in anticipating and avoiding the negative feedback (Gallagher & Reid, 1981; Montangero, 1985).

CONSTRUCTIVISM AND ADOLESCENT DEVELOPMENT

In this section, we characterize how these constructivist principles apply to adolescent development. Of course, this was articulated more than a half-century ago by Inhelder and Piaget (1958) in their account of the development of formal operations during adolescence. The book documents the emergence and consolidation of cognitive structures of formal operations (sixteen binary operations and the Identity, Negation, Reciprocity, and Correlativity group of transformations or the INRC group). In the book's last chapter, Inhelder and Piaget (1958) outline the consequences of formal operational thinking for adolescents' everyday thinking, feelings, and social relations. The uniqueness of this chapter in the broader work of Piaget is worth noting and was commented on by Flavell (1963, pp. 222–223) in his review of the theory: "As a rule, Piaget has been much more concerned with conceptualizing developmental change in cognitive structures per se than with trying to show how these changes are causally linked with changes in everyday cognitive, social, and affective behavior. It is therefore of interest that the book on adolescent reasoning concludes with a brief excursion of this type."

Noting that "there is more to thinking than logic," Inhelder and Piaget (1958, p. 335) explore changes in adolescent thinking, feeling, and social relationships as they move from puberty to the adoption of adult social roles. Biological changes in adolescents' bodies and brains serve as a context for adolescents' thinking about their future adult social roles. Such roles correspond to the sociological pressures to orient toward adulthood. But the chapter is notable for its focus not on biological or sociological factors but on the adolescent as an active agent of developmental change, seeking to understand and fit into the adult world. Although some of their account of teenage life seems dated (e.g., constructing *personal theories*, *life programs*, and *projects for changing the world*), Inhelder and Piaget (1958) describe adolescents as using their cognitive capacities to go beyond their immediate circumstances and project themselves into the adult social world. The account picks up the core constructivist view of adolescents as active agents using their cognitive powers in more or less conscious ways to make meaning of their circumstances and solve problems they encounter.

The constructivist account also recognizes inevitable vulnerabilities and opportunities as adolescents make sense of their world. Opportunities abound for adolescents whose self-constructed pathways to their own futures result in successful transitions into adulthood. But Inhelder and Piaget (1958) caution that more often than not, adolescents' visions of adulthood in general and their adulthood in particular are egocentric and immature, each reflecting a lack of adequate coordination. Adolescent egocentrism is the inevitable lack of understanding of the limits of new cognitive powers due to a lack of coordination with others' perspectives (also see Elkind, 1967). As a result, ideas are not well thought through beyond the sense they make to the adolescents themselves. Adolescent immaturity is the inevitable result of the slow process of acquiring new cognitive abilities. Early adolescence is a time of the initial emergence of formal operational thinking skills, but the skills are incompletely coordinated. The result is that young adolescents are able to entertain abstract and hypothetical ideas but are less capable of systematically testing them.

ON BABIES AND BATHWATER

In this section, we consider critiques of constructivist accounts of adolescent development and contend that, in these critiques, the constructivist baby has been thrown out with the Piagetian bathwater. As noted earlier, the Piagetian account of adolescent development has waned over the years. An accounting of articles in PSYCINFO containing the expression *formal*

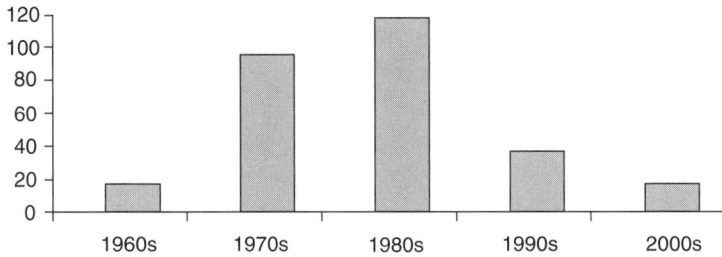

FIGURE 1.1. The frequency of peer-reviewed articles in PSYCINFO containing the expression *Formal Operations*, by decade.

operations reveals 289 separate articles in peer-reviewed journals. The distribution by decade of the number of these journal articles (Figure 1.1) indexes the rise and fall of research activity on interest in formal operations. As previously noted, mounting criticisms of the developmental diversity and plasticity in formal operational thinking were based on evidence of the contextual and cultural variation in such thinking.

Notwithstanding these criticisms and the resulting disinterest in studying formal operations, we review the constructivist approach here to reinvigorate the view of adolescence as a distinctive period of time in the life cycle of unique opportunities and vulnerabilities. This research focusing on the diversity and plasticity of development challenged Inhelder and Piaget's view of formal operations as being acquired exclusively (*de novo*) and completely (*in toto*) during adolescence. Research pointed to younger children's surprising demonstration of logical, hypothetical, and abstract thinking in certain domains, contexts, and cultures, as well as adolescents and adults' equally surprising failure to demonstrate such reasoning in other domains, contents, and cultures. All this seems to undermine the notion that a "stage" of formal operation was emerging spontaneously and universally. Among the abilities supposedly acquired uniquely by adolescents but demonstrated by children include scientific (see review by Zimmerman, 2000; 2007), logical reasoning (see review by Kuhn, 2009), moral reasoning (see reviews by Smetana, 2006; Turiel, 2006), and perspective taking (see review by Martin, Sokol, & Elfers, 2008). The abilities supposedly acquired uniquely by adolescents but *not* demonstrated by them or adults include rational judgment and decision making (see a review by Shaklee, 1979) and objective and systematic thinking (Amsel, Klaczynski, Johnston, Bench, Close, Sadler, & Walker, 2008).

In exploring what is distinctive in adolescent development, the authors in this volume focus on forms of adolescent *coordinating activities*. Many theories have long acknowledged that the developmental process involves connecting individual entities to other ones within a system or network, which increases the former's efficiency or effectiveness, such as its stability, control, power, or flexibility (c.f., Piaget, 1970; Vygotsky, 1962; Werner & Kaplan, 1963). By coordinating activities, we mean the integration of separate elements into an organized system of relations. This may occur at various levels of analysis, including connecting brain structures or processes into a neurological system; connecting cognitive elements such as capacities, beliefs, skills, or understandings into a conceptual structure; or connecting particular persons to others to create a social network. The new organized system of relations may become more efficient or effective in whatever function the individual elements were performing prior to their coordination. Again returning to the simple mathematical expressions, a sense of mathematical truth emerges when one procedure is coordinated with other ones in a set of related procedures. Despite the acquisition of each mathematical procedure, there is no grasp of the mathematical truth tapped by the procedures unless there is a coordination of them in an organized system.

As we discuss more fully later in the chapter, some coordinating activities create permanent connections between elements in the system, but in other cases the coordinating activity leads to temporary connections between elements that must be effectively reinstated in appropriate contexts. In either case, the new organization is a developmental transformation from the previous state of the organism, although all of the elements comprising the new organization were present earlier in development. The focus on adolescents' active coordination of preexisting elements suggests that adolescence changes are not *de novo* transformations, as the individual elements in the system may have existed prior to their coordination. Similarly, the focus on active coordinations that are temporary and need to be consistently reinstated by adolescents and adults suggests that adolescent changes are not *in toto* transformations, as they may extend into adulthood.

THEMES OF THE PAPERS

The book presents what we view as constructivist accounts of the adolescent coordinating activities in the domains of neurological structures and processes (Giedd and colleagues, Steinberg), cognitive systems (Amsel, Steinberg), cognitive strategies and metacognitive processes (Kuhn & Holman), experiences and self-narratives (Thorne & Shapiro), social reasoning and parental relations (Smetana), understanding of and interactions with friends (Bukowski, Simard, Dubois, & Lopez), and relations between self and the broader developmental ecology (Crosnoe). Although the domains are quite distinct, each account presumes that adolescents make sense of their world through coordinating activities that shape their own development.

We review each contribution with an eye to highlighting the constructivist aspects that each author incorporates in his or her view of adolescent development. To this end, we highlight each contribution not only for the forms of coordination within levels or planes of analysis (neurological, cognitive, and social), but also between these levels, including the neurological and cognitive levels (Giedd and colleagues, Steinberg), cognitive and social levels (Amsel, Bukowsky et al., Crosnoe, Smetana, Steinberg, Thorne & Shapiro), and neurological and social levels (Steinberg). Additionally, adolescents' coordinating activities are explored in terms of opportunities for positive developmental outcomes they provide and vulnerabilities they pose if these coordinations are unsuccessful. These outcomes include the impact of unsuccessful coordinations for adolescent well-being (Bukowski et al.), mental health (Giedd, Crosnoe), risk taking (Steinberg, Amsel), parental conflict (Smetana), and academic underachievement (Kuhn & Holman, Crosnoe).

Biological and Cognitive Development

Giedd and colleagues present a broad description of neurological changes in cortical and subcortical regions from childhood to adolescence. They also summarize important new work exploring the genetic and environmental contributions to those brain changes based on the longitudinal twin study Giedd has been leading over the past several years. Many of the brain changes across neurological subdivisions appear to be inherited, suggesting that these changes were evolutionarily shaped and genetically mediated. Against this background, Giedd and colleagues report that there are dynamic changes in the heritability of neurological changes across ages. The volume of white matter in the brain lobes grows linearly and becomes more strongly associated with additive genetic contribution over age, whereas the volume of gray matter, which grows in an "inverted U"-shaped trajectory, becomes more strongly associated with unique environmental contributions over age.

Giedd and colleagues note that brain mechanisms responsible for the neural reorganization of white and gray matter is more coordinated and connected than it may appear, with a few dedicated mechanisms being implicated. They acknowledge that myelinization has been thought to under-lie the increase of white matter in the adolescent brain. However, recent work suggests that the change may be due to a speeding up of neurotrans-mission-related machinery in the axon (Giorgio, Watkins, Chadwick, James, Winmill, et al., 2010; Paus, 2010), which may also be influenced by envi-ronmental factors, including learning (Fields, 2008a, 2008b). Whatever the underlying mechanism, white matter increase is associated with improve-ments in the timing and flow of information between neurons.

Giedd and colleagues also note that changes in cortical gray matter may be due to processes of synaptic overproduction (synaptic blooming) and elimination (synaptic pruning) and to the myelinization of intracor-tical axons. Although the researchers do not offer an explanation of the increasing unique environmental contributions to the changes in gray mat-ter over age, it may be related to the later synaptic pruning process, which is more dependent on experience than the earlier synaptic blooming process (Huttenlocher, 1994, although see Paus, 2005, 2009). Again, whatever the process, gray matter changes during adolescence, particularly in the pre-frontal cortex, are associated with increased efficiency, effectiveness, and control of brain function (Casey, Jones, & Hare, 2008; Paus, 2005, 2009).

Giedd and colleagues make clear how the shaping of the brain during adolescence creates potential opportunities for positive developmental outcomes and vulnerabilities to more negative ones. The age x heritabil-ity findings suggest that normal developmental trajectories depend on the appropriate timing of the expression of particular genes to initiate brain reorganization; otherwise the adolescent is susceptible to the emergence of a range of mental health disorders. However, critical to this discussion, the normal trajectory of brain maturation during adolescence makes for faster, more efficient, and better controlled neural activity, resulting in adolescents having greater opportunities to coordinate neurological networks. That is, the evolutionarily shaped, genetically mediated, and environmentally impacted mechanisms of brain sculpting create a neurological platform in which opportunities for active coordinations between neurological systems become more available to adolescents, as compared to children.

Steinberg's chapter continues the focus on changes in adolescent brain function and organization to predict important cognitive changes with which they may be associated. He articulates an account of two relatively distinct neurological networks – the "socioemotional" and "cognitive con-trol" systems – and highlights their normal trajectory of development. The socioemotional system is activated through puberty-related mechanisms during early adolescence and is associated with increases in reward-seeking behavior. The maturation of the cognitive control system, with its executive control functions, is related to independent pruning and myelinization processes that occur later in adolescent development.

Over time, there is increased connectivity between the systems, which enables them to function together, thereby improving the cognitive control over and regulation of affect. The growth of connectivity represents a form of active coordination central to a constructivist account of adolescent development. There is reason to think that this coordination is related to adolescents' own activities and experiences (Fields, 2008a, 2008b; Giedd, 2004). However, the asynchrony of the timing between the maturation of these systems is the focus of Steinberg's chapter. He presents evidence of the dual-system model by testing the novel distinction between reward seeking (which, as a socio-emotional function, should peak in early adolescence) and impulse control (which, as a cognitive control function, should peak in later adolescence). He finds support for his predictions, suggesting a distinct vulnerability for young adolescents whose reward sensitivity and inclinations may be unchecked by an immaturely developed system for exercising executive control over impulses. Steinberg draws out the consequences of this vulnerability for the risk-seeking activities of some young adolescents, but it might be equally applied to the risk-avoiding activities of other adolescents (Reyna & Farley, 2006), or even both activities in same adolescents who may actively seek out some risks and avoid others (Shaw, Amsel, & Schilo, in press). Behavior is channeled into activities that bring social or material rewards without any deeper considerations of the implications, consequences, or justifications of such actions.

Steinberg presents his work as a form of contextualism which highlights adolescent development as a product of the complex interaction of forces in teenagers' bio-ecology. For example, he reviews evidence repudiating explanations of adolescent risk-taking that take a cognitive developmental perspective and the effectiveness of risk-taking interventions designed to promote adolescent cognitive development. His concluding remarks imply that young adolescents' behavior can be best regulated not by promoting cognitive changes which are constrained by neurological immaturity, but by changing the contexts in which they find themselves.

Despite the constraint of neurological immaturity, adolescents may nonetheless construct new ways of thinking, reasoning, and understanding to cope with and comprehend the puberty-related changes they are undergoing. Thus, the cognitive changes during adolescence may be encouraged by changes in adolescents' social context rather than being seen as constrained by the process of neurological maturation. This point was made from a constructivist perspective by Inhelder and Piaget (1958, p. 337) in the last chapter of the *Growth of Logical Thinking from Childhood to Adolescence.*

> In sum, far from being a source of fully elaborated "innate ideas," the maturation of the nervous system can do no more than determine the totality of possibilities and impossibilities at a given stage. A particular social environment remains indispensible in the realization of these possibilities. It follows that their realization can be accelerated or retarded as a function of cultural and educational conditions.

The central role of education in adolescent cognitive development is the focus of the chapter by Kuhn and Holman. The chapter highlights a number of skills central to the effective functioning of adolescents in the twenty-first century and the forms of curricular interventions necessary to promote them. The prescribed skill set for optimal cognitive functioning involves coordinating activities between (a) multiple variables, levels within variables, and evidence bearing on each variable in complex causal contexts; (b) multiple perspectives and their strengths and weaknesses in dialogic argument contexts; and (c) general cognitive and epistemological principles or dispositions and an array of cognitive strategies and processes they ought to govern across different contexts. Coordinating activities are further needed to relate these skills to one another to arm adolescents with a competent, persistent, and multifaceted approach to argumentation.

Kuhn and Holman's description of the curriculum needed to promote these skills highlights how active coordinations can be directed to improve reasoning. The curriculum, designed for middle school students, is embedded in naturalistic argumentative activities (debates), which are extended over time. The three forms of coordinating activities are authentically enhanced in the curriculum by the use of argument topics of interest to participants who, together with partners, prepare, state, and evaluate arguments defending their own and attacking others' positions. The curriculum is shown to be effective at each level of analysis – argument recognition, evidence integration, strategic transfer across topics and formats (oral vs. written), and metacognitive development – which Kuhn and Holman note ironically includes a decrease in certainty in their positions as participants learn to readily anticipate other positions than their own.

It would seem that multiple levels of cognitive development, from the acquisition of specific strategies to broad metacognitive skills, are central to coordinating activities that promote stable intellectual growth. This is also the message of Amsel's chapter, which examines the development of hypothetical thinking during adolescence. Amsel traces skills for hypothetical thinking to the fanciful pretend play activities of young children. Pretending children behave with respect to representations of alternative pretend worlds which parallel but are distinct and distinguished from representations of the world that are believed to be true. Amsel argues that coordinating activities in the form of metacognitive evaluation and executive control are necessary for fanciful pretend worlds to become serious possible ones. These coordinating activities are acquired slowly over childhood and adolescence, and their timing appears asynchronous over different contexts where hypothetical thinking is used. Moreover, coordinating activities in the form of relating real and possible worlds, including subordinating the latter to the former emphasized by Inhelder and Piaget as a core acquisition in adolescence, are also slowly acquired and remain a challenge for adults in some contexts. Although component skills necessary for hypothetical thinking may be available in childhood, it is not until adolescence that the range of relevant knowledge, strategies, metacognitive processes, and executive control are actively coordinated so they can work together in the service of hypothetical thinking. The expertise at hypothetical reasoning develops as adolescents gain practice in coordinating these skills.

Amsel proposes a dual-process model of the development of hypothetical thinking which emphasizes the coordination between two cognitive systems – automatic, spontaneous, and largely unconscious *experiential* processes, on the one hand, and effortful, systematic, and largely conscious *analytic* processes, on the other. Experiential processes for creating alternative worlds are coordinated with analytic ones for transforming representations of alternative worlds into possible ones and comparing possible to actual ones. The dual cognitive systems Amsel proposes share some similarities with the dual neurological systems articulated by Steinberg. Both propose a developmental trajectory emphasizing the coordination between systems rather than the dominance of one system over another. The connections between the two systems in Steinberg's model become permanently rewired, ensuring the potential of their coordination. But this is not so for Amsel's dual-process model, which requires constant metacognitive monitoring and regulation of the two systems which may vary by contexts and over people.

Neurological development during adolescence makes possible but also may be shaped by coordinating activities of adolescents. The reshaped neurological platform enables adolescents to coordinate various cognitive entities and processes and construct new abilities, including those for argumentation and hypothetical thinking. These abilities are both opportunities for adolescents as argumentation and hypothetical thinking reflect forms of mature thinking. But there are not only cognitive, but also psychosocial and social-relational vulnerabilities for adolescents who fail to engage in the forms of coordinating activities necessary for constructing such skills. Steinberg identifies one form of resultant cognitive immaturity as lack of impulse control (as distinguished from risk-seeking behavior), which may make it difficult for adolescents to form healthy social relationships. Kuhn and Holman suggest that academic underachievement and missed social opportunities are consequences of failure to engage in coordinating activities leading to the development of argument skills. Similarly, Amsel notes that the cognitive immaturity resulting from the failure to engage in forms of coordinating activities resulting in hypothetical thinking may affect adolescents' mental health and social relations.

Psychosocial and Socio-Relational Development

The coordinating activities in the four chapters addressing psychosocial and socio-relational development in some cases have a very different form than the coordinating activities at the neurological and cognitive levels. Psychosocial and socio-relational coordinating activities are between an individual and others, including friends, parents, social networks of peers, or even oneself. Thorne and Shapiro make the latter point clear in their discussion of the narrative account of identity development. A careful read of their chapter reveals forms of cognitive coordinating activities in the development of self-narratives, including hypothetical reasoning (adopting others' perspectives) and argument skills (defending against others' (mis) interpretations of shared narratives). They also highlight a social form of coordinating activities between the self as narrator (William James' *I*), and the self as experience (James' *me*), whose past and present experiences must be merged into a coherent narrative. Social coordinating activities are also found in relating one's own story to grand narratives of the broader culture. Finally, parent-child interactions that scaffold and spiral dialogues about the self are also discussed as social coordinating activities which promote the construction of identity narratives.

While these narratives may not be permanent identities, stable over time and space, they are important elements of the self that are publically tested and privately held to shape future experiences. Thorne and Shapiro's emphasis on how adolescents and young adults test their identities through storytelling highlights yet another form of socially-based coordinating activities: Those between the person and the audience. The audience to whom a story about the self is being told is critical in the construction of self-narratives because, as Thorne and Shapiro remind us, the story told is as well remembered as the experience lived. The reaction of the audience helps the storyteller in interpreting the meaning of lived experiences. Thorne and Shapiro highlight the importance of selecting an appropriate audience to test a self narrative so as to shape its meaning.

Smetana's chapter underscores the coordinating processes leading adolescents to construct new social-cognitive understandings and social relationships. She examines adolescent-parent relationships as a context for studying social-cognitive and socio-relational development, asking why adolescent-parent conflict increases and closeness decreases. She proposes that the relationship transforms as conflicts increase over the scope and boundaries of various social domains. These domains include a *personal* sense of control, privacy, and preferences; *social* worlds of norms, expectations, and authorities; *moral* prescriptions regarding fairness, obligation, and rights; and *prudential* concerns about health, safety, and happiness. As adolescents carve out a personal space in which to explore themselves and their potential, the scope of their personal domain expands ("It is my choice to. . . ."). But as the adolescent's personal domain expands, it crosses parental boundaries of the social, moral, and/ or prudential domain, igniting their expression of authority ("As your Mom, I can't let you. . . .").

Smetana reports on the development of processes for coordinating these domains within individual adolescents and between adolescents and their parents. Adolescents coordinate the relations between these social domains by altering the demarcation between them. As suggested above, the domain of personal control, privacy and, preferences expands over adolescence as they perform the identity work that is triggered by puberty. This coordinating activity between the realms of identity development and the scope of the personal domain is unique to adolescence. Smetana further suggests that parent–adolescent conflict is an effective way for adolescents to negotiate this expanding autonomy with parents. Peers are also implicated in this negotiation process as they offer norms about what can be expected by way of autonomy over the personal domain. Less effective negotiating strategies include teens withholding information, which, although minimizing conflict, may be associated with other problems. However, it is the parents' expectations about their adolescents' autonomy that predicts their level of later autonomy over the personal domain. Smetana concludes that coordinating activities which relate social domains (such as the personal and prudential) to each other can also be used to harmonize social domains between parents and adolescents to reduce conflict and improve the relationship.

Bukowski, Simard, Dubois, and Lopez also emphasize the role of adolescents' cognitive and social coordinating activities in their construction of new understandings and relationships. They explore these processes in the domain of friendship in early adolescence. Bukowski et al. review classic research on adolescents' conceptions of friendship. They point out that adolescents' notion of friendship become increasing psychological and relational as they focus on such components as companionship, conflict, help, security, and closeness. These forms of social interactions or social exchanges are subject to further coordinating activities by adolescents as they create an internalized representation of a meaningful emotional relationship with a targeted other. Indeed, adolescents may be at risk if they fail to engage in the coordinating activities that transform behavioral interactions into representations of friendships.

Bukowski et al. report the results of longitudinal research testing their model of friendship development. The findings confirm that the number of quality interactions in early adolescence predict later friendships, and that the friendships but not the interactions, are related to adolescents' well-being. Moreover, the relationship between interactions and friendships was found for middle-socioeconomic status (SES) adolescents, but not for the highest or lowest SES groups, whose interactions with companions were not represented as intimate friends. Bukowski et al. conclude that the study of the process of friendship formation must go beyond the focus on elementary behaviors indexing particular social interactions to the study of more coordinated representations of friendships.

The notion that development is promoted by social coordinating activities between adolescents and parents or friends can also be extended to adolescents' coordinating activities with peer networks. Crosnoe's chapter highlights how such coordinating activities can promote or derail positive developmental trajectories. Crosnoe explores adolescent peer relations in high school, which is much more salient to teens as a social than an educational context. He examines how the social coordination of adolescents with their high school peers can influence their academic trajectory. The focus of his work is on adolescents stigmatized by obesity or poverty and socially marginalized because of it. Typically these students' short-term coping strategies (e.g., disengagement, negative self-image, and self-medication) are counterproductive as they result in a negative long-term academic trajectory.

Crosnoe tested a model of the mediating effect of school culture on the academic trajectory of stigmatized adolescent youth. That is, he asked whether the effects of stigmatization on obese and poor adolescents' academic trajectories would be mitigated by whether their school is a "heavy" or "poor" one? He found a moderating effect for social group dynamics, particularly for girls. College participation for obese girls was higher for girls in schools that were above rather than below the national average for weight. Similarly college attendance was higher for poor girls in schools in which most parents were not college educated (an index of SES) than those in schools with mostly college-educated parents. The implication of the data is that adolescent social coordination with their high school peer culture mediates their short-term social development and long-term academic preparation. Crosnoe concludes that this process reflects adolescents agentive social nature in trying to understand where they fit socially and in managing the consequences of not doing so. But in the modern large, impersonal, and diverse high school, where older traditional and newer digital modes of communication can be used as a weapon to communicate difference, stigmatized adolescents' academic trajectories may become more vulnerable depending on their school's culture.

SUMMARY AND CONCLUSIONS

The goal of this book is to reassert a constructivist approach to adolescent development with the image of adolescents as *architects* whose activities drive their own development. We have highlighted the importance of considering adolescents' coordinating activities, which involve linking elementary processes, structures, and individuals together at the neurological, cognitive, and social levels. These activities are shown to afford opportunities for positive developmental outcomes and vulnerabilities for less positive outcomes.

Our focus on adolescents' coordinating activities is *not* a prelude for a new broad-based theory of adolescent development in the tradition of other grand developmental theories (see Amsel & Renninger, 1997). Rather, we highlight adolescents' coordinating activities as a strategy for researchers and theorists to identify processes across a range of domains that are consistent with a constructivist account of adolescent development. As we see it, opportunities to identify and elaborate accounts of adolescent coordinating activities have been overlooked, leaving unexplored potentially fruitful new research directions focusing on neurological, cognitive and social development realized by such activities. We invite readers to carefully review the chapters and discover for themselves the parallels that exist across the range of insightful accounts of adolescent development in the present collection.

ACKNOWLEDGMENTS

We are grateful to Cecilia Wainryb for helpful comments on this chapter.

REFERENCES

Amsel, E., Klaczynski, P. A., Johnston, A., Bench, S., Close, J., Sadler, E., & Walker, R. (2008). A dual-process account of the development of scientific reasoning: The nature and development of metacognitive intercession skills. *Cognitive Development, 23*, 451–471.

Amsel, E., & Renninger, K. A. (Eds.). (1997). *Change and development: Issues of theory, method and application.* Mahwah, NJ: Lawrence Erlbaum Associates.

Casey, B. J., Jones, R. M., & Hare, T. A. (2008). The adolescent brain. *Annals of New York Academy of Sciences, 1124*, 111–126.

Elkind, D. (1967). Egocentrism in adolescence. *Child Development, 38*, 1025–1034.

Erikson, E. H. (1968). *Identity: Youth and crisis.* New York: Norton.

Fields, R. D. (2008a). White matter in learning, cognition and psychiatric disorders. *Trends in Neuroscience, 31*, 361–370.

     (2008b). White matter matters. *Scientific American, 298*, 42–49.

Flavell, J. (1963). *The developmental psychology of Jean Piaget.* New York: Van Nostrand Reinhold.

Gallagher, J., & Reid, D. (1981). *The learning theory of Piaget and Inhelder.* Austin, TX: Pro-Ed.

Giedd, J. (2004). Structural magnetic resonance imaging of the adolescent brain. Annals of the *New York Academy of Sciences, 1021*, 77–85.

Giorgio, K. E., Watkins, M., Chadwick, S., James, L., Winmill, G., et al. (2010). Longitudinal changes in grey and white matter during adolescence. *NeuroImage, 49*, 94–103.

Huttenlocher, P. R. (1994). Synaptogenesis, synapse elimination, and neural plasticity in human cerebral cortex. In C. A. Nelson (Ed.), *Threats to optimal development: The Minnesota symposia on child psychology: Vol. 27* (pp. 35–54). Hillsdale, NJ: Lawrence Erlbaum.

Inhelder, I., & Piaget, J. (1958). *The growth of logical thinking from childhood to adolescence.* New York: Basic Books.

Kohlberg, L. (1969). Stage and sequence: The cognitive developmental approach to socialization. In D. Goslin (Ed.), *Handbook of socialization theory and research* (pp. 347–480). Chicago: Rand McNally.

Kuhn, D. (2009). Adolescent thinking. In R. Lerner & L. Steinberg (Eds.), *Handbook of adolescent psychology* (3rd ed., Vol. 1, pp. 152–186). New York: Wiley.

Langer, J. (1969). *Theories of development.* New York: Holt, Reinhart, & Winston.

Lerner, R., & Steinberg, L. (2009). The scientific study of adolescence: Past, present, and future. In R. Lerner and L. Steinberg (Eds.), *Handbook of adolescent psychology* (3rd ed., Vol. 1., pp. 3–14). New York: Wiley.

Martin, J., Sokol, B. W., & Elfers, T. (2008). Taking and coordinating perspectives: From prereflective interactivity, through reflective intersubjectivity, to metareflective sociality. *Human Development, 51,* 294–317.

Montangero, J. (1985). *Genetic epistemology yesterday and today.* New York: The Graduate School and City University of New York.

Moshman, D. (2005). *Adolescent psychological development: Rationality, morality, and identity* (2nd ed.), Mahwah, NJ: Lawrence Erlbaum Associates.

Paus, T. (2005). Mapping brain maturation and cognitive development during adolescence. *Trends in Cognitive Science, 9,* 60–68.

(2009). Brain development. In R. Lerner & L. Steinberg (Eds.), *Handbook of adolescent psychology* (3rd ed., Vol 1., pp. 95–115). New York: Wiley.

(2010). Growth of white matter in the adolescent brain: Myelin or axon? *Brain and Cognition, 72,* 26–35.

Piaget, J. (1970). Piaget's theory. In P. H. Mussen (Ed.), *Carmichael's manual of child psychology* (Vol. 1, pp. 103–128). New York: Wiley.

Reese, H. W., & Overton W. F. (1970). Models of development and theories of development. In L. R. Goulet & R. B. Baltes (Eds.), *Life-span developmental psychology: Research and theory* (pp. 116–145). New York: Academic Press.

Reyna, V. F., & Farley, F. (2006). Risk and rationality in adolescent decision making: Implications for theory, practice, and public policy. *Psychological Science in the Public Interest, 7,* 1–44.

Shaklee, H. (1979). Bounded rationality and cognitive development: Upper limits on growth? *Cognitive Psychology, 11,* 327–345.

Shaw, L., Amsel, E., & Schilo, J. (in press). Risk taking in late adolescence: Relations between socio-moral reasoning, risk stance and behavior. *Journal of Research in Adolescence.*

Smetana, J. G. (2006). Social domain theory: Consistencies and variations in children's moral and social judgments. In M. Killen & J. G. Smetana (Eds.), *Handbook of moral development* (pp. 119–154). Mahwah, NJ: Erlbaum.

Turiel, E. (2006). The development of morality. In N. Eisenberg, W. Damon, & R. M. Lerner (Eds.), *Handbook of child psychology: Social, emotional, and personality development* (pp. 789–857). Hoboken, NJ: Wiley.

Vygotsky, L. S. (1962). *Thought and language.* Cambridge, MA: MIT Press.

Werner, H., & Kaplan, B. (1963). *Symbol formation: An organismic-developmental approach to language and the expression of thought.* New York: Wiley.

Zimmerman, C. (2000). The development of scientific reasoning skills. *Developmental Review, 20,* 99–149.

Zimmerman, C. (2007). The development of scientific thinking skills in elementary and middle school. *Developmental Review, 27,* 172–223.

PART I

BIOLOGICAL AND COGNITIVE PERSPECTIVE

2

Structural Brain Magnetic Resonance Imaging of Typically Developing Children and Adolescents

JAY N. GIEDD, ARMIN RAZNAHAN, NANCY R. LEE,
CATHERINE WEDDLE, MARIA LIVERPOOL, MICHAEL
STOCKMAN, ELIZABETH M. WELLS, LIV CLASEN,
JONATHAN BLUMENTHAL, RHOSHEL K.
LENROOT, AND FRANCOIS LALONDE
Child Psychiatry Branch, National Institute of Mental Health

Magnetic resonance imaging (MRI) provides unprecedented access to the anatomy and physiology of the human brain and has launched a new era of pediatric neuroscience. Because it does not use ionizing radiation, it is safe not only for single scans of children, but for repeated scans throughout the course of maturation. In this chapter, we will summarize results to date from an ongoing longitudinal brain MRI project that has been underway at the Child Psychiatry Branch (CPB) of the National Institute of Mental Health (NIMH) since being initiated by Dr. Markus Krusei in 1989. The design of the study is for volunteers to visit the NIMH at approximately two-year intervals for (1) genetic analysis; (2) cognitive/emotional/behavioral assessment; and (3) brain imaging.

The data presented here are the quantitative morphology (i.e., size and shape) results from our typically developing participants between the ages of three and twenty-seven years. The findings will be grouped by tissue type (i.e., gray matter, white matter, cerebrospinal fluid) or structure/region (i.e. total and lobar volumes, caudate, ventricles, etc.) and shown as a function of age separately for boys and girls. To promote independence of the sample data points for the non-twin analyses, only one subject was chosen per family. The particular person chosen from a given family was based on an attempt to optimize the age and gender distribution of the sample and was done blind to knowledge of their imaging results. Unless otherwise indicated, the results in the following sections are from the most recent analyses of the CPB data consisting of 829 scans from 387 subjects, ages 3 to 27 years.

TRAJECTORIES OF BRAIN MORPHOMETRY IN TYPICAL PEDIATRIC DEVELOPMENT

Total Cerebral Volume

In the CPB cohort, total cerebral volume peaks at 10.5 years in females and 14.5 years in males (Lenroot et al., 2007). By age six years, the brain is at approximately 95 percent of this peak (see Figure 2.1). That total cerebral volume decreases during adolescence was not previously detected with postmortem data (Dekaban, 1977; Dekaban and Sadowsky, 1978) or cross-sectional MRI studies (Jernigan and Tallal, 1990; Giedd, Snell, et al., 1996). Consistent with previous reports (Goldstein et al., 2001), mean total cerebral volume is approximately 10 percent larger in males. Total brain size differences should not be interpreted as imparting any sort of functional advantage or disadvantage. Gross structural measures may not reflect sexually dimorphic differences in functionally relevant factors such as neuronal connectivity and receptor density. Of note is the high variability of brain size even in this group of rigorously screened children and adolescents who were healthy. Children who were healthy and normally functioning at the same age may have as much as a 50 percent difference in total brain volume, further highlighting the need to be cautious regarding functional implications of absolute brain sizes.

Ventricles

Consistent with previous reports of greater ventricular volume in adults versus children (Jernigan and Tallal, 1990), lateral ventricular volume increased robustly with age in the CPB sample of children and adolescents who were healthy (see Figure 2.1d). This is noteworthy because increased ventricular volumes are associated with a broad range of neuropsychiatric conditions. That ventricular volume is highly variable, and increases in healthy pediatric development, complicates interpretation of ventricular volume changes in patient populations.

White Matter

Magnetic resonance imaging voxels containing a sufficient amount of myelinated axons are classified as WM. Myelination is the wrapping of oligodendrocytes around axons that increases the speed of neuronal signal transmission and modulates the timing and synchrony of neuronal firing patterns that convey meaning in the brain (Fields and Stevens-Graham, 2002).

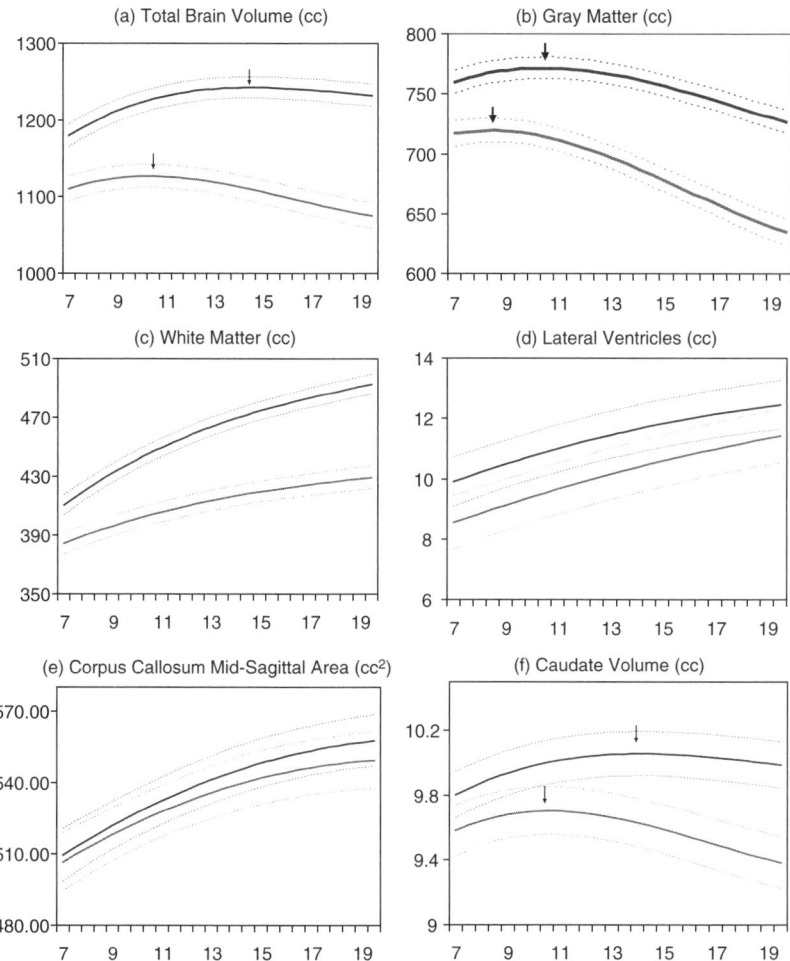

FIGURE 2.1. Mean volume by age in years for males ($N = 475$ scans) and females ($N = 354$ scans). Middle lines in each set of three lines represent mean values, and upper and lower lines represent upper and lower 95% confidence intervals. All curves differed significantly in height and shape with the exception of lateral ventricles, in which only height was different, and mid-sagittal area of the corpus callosum, in which neither height nor shape was different. (a) Total brain volume, (b) gray matter volume, (c) white matter volume, (d) lateral ventricle volume, (e) mid-sagittal area of the corpus callosum, and (f) caudate volume.

Consistent with previous reports (Pfefferbaum et al., 1994; Giedd et al., 1995; Reiss et al., 1996; Giedd, Blumenthal, Jeffries, Castellanos, et al., 1999; Giedd, Blumenthal, Jeffries, Rajapakse, et al., 1999; Sowell et al., 2001; Sowell et al., 2003; Lenroot et al., 2007), WM volumes increase throughout childhood and adolescence (see Figure 2.1c). The rate of increase is age-dependent

(Giedd, Blumenthal, Jeffries, Castellanos, et al., 1999) and can increase as much as 50 percent in small regions of interest (Thompson et al., 2000), but at the lobar level (frontal, temporal, and parietal lobes), developmental WM trajectories are similar.

The most prominent WM structure is the corpus callosum (CC) consisting of approximately 200 million axons connecting homologous areas of the left and right cortex. The organization of the CC is roughly topographic, with anterior, middle, and posterior segments containing fibers from their corresponding cortical regions. The functions of the CC can generally be thought of as integrating the activities of the left and right cerebral hemispheres, including functions related to the unification of sensory fields (Shanks et al., 1975; Berlucchi, 1981), memory storage and retrieval (Zaidel and Sperry, 1974), attention and arousal (Levy, 1985), and enhancement of language and auditory functions (Cook, 1986). The relationship between improved capacities for these functions during childhood and adolescence and the noted morphologic changes is intriguing. Several studies have indicated that CC development continues to progress throughout adolescence (Allen et al., 1991; Cowell et al., 1992; Pujol et al., 1993; Rauch and Jinkins, 1994; Thompson et al., 2000), raising the question of whether this may be related to the improvement in these cognitive capacities seen during childhood and adolescence. In the CPB sample, total mid-sagittal CC area increased robustly from ages four to twenty years (see Figure 2.1e).

The growing interest in exploring neural circuitry has encouraged the development of newer MR techniques, such as magnetization transfer (MT) imaging and diffusion tensor imaging (DTI), which allow characterization of the microstructure of WM and the direction of axons. These techniques have begun to be applied to pediatric populations.

DTI studies of typical child and adolescent development have consistently shown decreases of overall diffusion and increases in anisotropy (a measure of the directionality or nonrandomness of the diffusion; see Cascio et al., 2007, for review). High anisotropy measures are thought to reflect coherently bundled myelinated axons and axonal pruning (Suzuki et al., 2003) that allow greater efficiency of neuronal communication.

A growing body of literature documents a relationship between anisotropy measures and cognitive abilities. In a study of twenty-three healthy subjects aged seven to eighteen years, high anisotropy in the temporal lobe correlated with memory capacity and high anisotropy in the frontal lobe correlated with language ability (Nagy et al., 2004). High anisotropy in frontal and occipitoparietal association areas correlated with intelligence quotient (IQ) in a DTI study of forty-seven healthy subjects aged five to eighteen years (Schmithorst et al., 2005). A positive correlation between anisotropy in temporal and parietal areas and reading ability has been reported in three pediatric DTI studies (Beaulieu et al., 2005; Deutsch et al., 2005; Niogi and McCandliss, 2006). A DTI study of twenty-one subjects, aged seven to thirty-one years, demonstrated decreased diffusion of WM fibers connecting the ventral prefrontal cortex to the caudate nucleus, which was paralleled by improvements in reaction time and cognitive performance (Liston et al., 2006).

MT imaging relates the number of protons bound to macromolecules to the number of unbound (free) protons, reflected as the magnetization transfer ratio (MTR) (Rovaris et al., 2003). MTR values are decreased with demyelination or axonal loss (Brochet and Dousset, 1999) and increase with myelination. Studies of children and adolescents who are healthy have reported MTR values increasing with maturation (Engelbrecht et al., 1998; van Buchem et al., 2001; Mukherjee and McKinstry, 2006), although the only study linking MTR values to cognitive performance thus far has been in adults (Lee et al., 2004).

Gray Matter

The composition of MRI voxels classified as GM may vary by region but by default these are voxels with not enough myelin to be classified as WM or enough fluid to be classified as cerebrospinal fluid (CSF). Unlike WM, during childhood and adolescence GM trajectories follow an inverted *U*-shaped path with total GM peaking at age 8.5 years in females and 10.5 years in males (see Figure 2.1b). This decoupling of developmental curves for GM and WM belies the inseparable connection among neurons, glial cells, and myelin, which are fellow components in neural circuits and are bound by lifelong reciprocal relationships (Fields and Stevens-Graham, 2002).

Cortical Gray Matter

At the lobar level, age at attainment of peak volumes of cortical GM varies by region and generally occurs earlier in girls. Thus, GM volumes peak in the frontal lobes at 9.5 years in girls and 10.5 years in boys, in the temporal lobes at 10.0 years in girls and 11.0 years in boys, and in the parietal lobes at 7.5 years in girls and 9 years in boys (see Figure 2.2).

To assess cortical GM at greater spatial resolution, we examined change in GM from ages four to twenty years on a voxel-by-voxel basis in a group of thirteen subjects who had each been scanned four times at approximately two-year intervals (Gogtay et al., 2004). An animation of these changes is

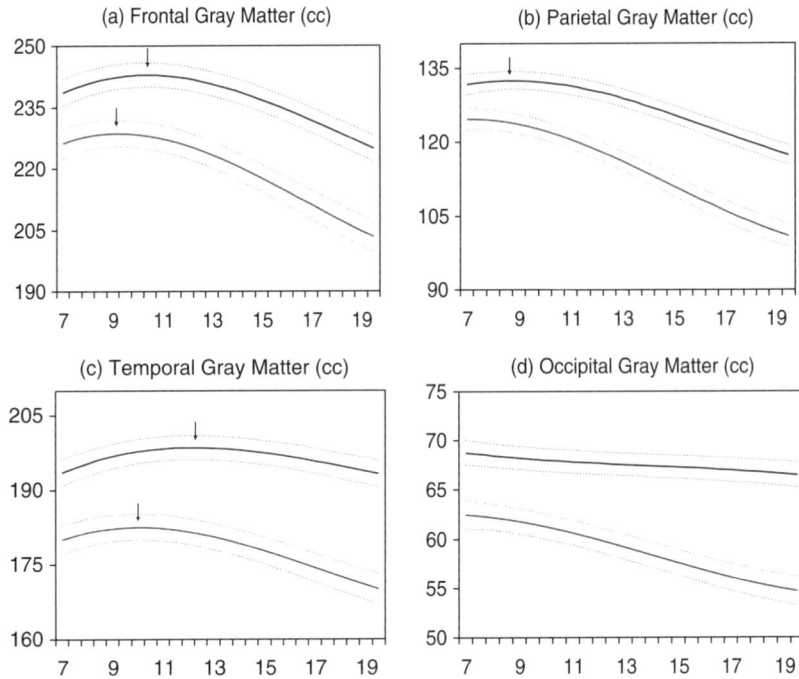

FIGURE 2.2. Gray matter subdivisions: (a) frontal lobe, (b) parietal lobe, (c) temporal lobe, and (d) occipital lobe.

available at http://www.loni.ucla.edu/~thompson/DEVEL/dyanamic.html. As with the lobar measurements, childhood GM increase is followed by loss beginning at different ages in different regions. Cortical GM loss occurs earliest in the primary sensorimotor areas and latest in the dorsolateral pre-frontal cortex (DLPFC), inferior parietal, and superior temporal gyrus. Areas subserving primary functions, such as motor and sensory systems, mature earliest. Higher-order association areas that integrate those pri-mary functions mature later. For example, the late-maturing superior tem-poral gyrus (along with prefrontal and inferior parietal cortices) serves as a heteromodal association site integrating memory, audio-visual input, and object recognition functions (Mesulam, 1998; Calvert, 2001; Martin and Chao, 2001).

Elucidating the cellular events underlying the GM volume changes is an area of active inquiry in neuroimaging research. Postmortem studies sug-gest that part of the GM changes may be related to synaptic proliferation and pruning (Huttenlocher, 1994). A study acquiring MRI and quantified elec-troencephalogram (EEG) in 138 healthy subjects aged 10 to 30 years found curvilinear reductions in frontal and parietal GM were matched by similar curvilinear reductions in EEG power of the corresponding regions, supporting the connection between GM volume reductions, EEG changes, and synaptic pruning (Whitford et al., 2007). Myelination may change classification of voxels along the interior cortical border from GM to WM, resulting in cortical thinning as assessed by MR volumetrics, without necessarily entailing changes in synaptic density (Sowell et al., 2001). Knowledge of the degree to which these and other phenomena may be driving the MR changes has profound implications for interpreting the imaging results. Imaging of nonhuman primates with postmortem validation may help in this regard.

Subcortical Gray Matter

BASAL GANGLIA. The basal ganglia are a collection of subcortical nuclei that are involved in circuits mediating movement, higher cognitive functions, attention, and affective states. Anomalous volumes of basal ganglia structures have been reported for almost all neuropsychiatric disorders that have been investigated by neuroimaging (Giedd et al., 2006). The basal ganglia comprise the caudate, putamen, globus pallidus, subthalamic nucleus, and substantia nigra. Because of the small size and ambiguity of MR signal contrast of the borders defining the structures, only the first three are readily quantifiable by MRI, and automated techniques have only been established as reliable for measurement of the caudate. Like the cortical GM structures, the caudate nucleus follows an inverted *U*-shape developmental trajectory. Caudate size peaks at age 10.5 years in girls and 14.0 years in boys (see Figure 2.1f). The shape of the caudate developmental trajectory is more similar to that of frontal and parietal GM than temporal. This supports the notion that brain regions that share extensive connections also share similar developmental courses.

AMYGDALA AND HIPPOCAMPUS. The temporal lobes, amygdala, and hippocampus are integral players in the arenas of emotion, language, and memory (Nolte, 1993). Human capacity for these functions changes markedly between the ages of four and eighteen years (Jerslid, 1963; Wechsler, 1974; Diener et al., 1985), although the relationship between the development of these capacities and morphological changes in the structures subserving these functions is poorly understood.

The amygdala and hippocampus have not been quantified for the longitudinal sample. In a previous report from a cross-sectional subset of the NIMH sample, amygdala volume increased significantly only in males, and hippocampal volume increased significantly with age only in females (Giedd, Vaituzis, et al., 1996). This pattern of gender-specific maturational volumetric changes is consistent with nonhuman primate studies indicating a relatively high number of androgen receptors in the amygdala (Clark et al., 1988) and a relatively higher number of estrogen receptors in the hippocampus (Morse et al., 1986), although direct links between receptor density and growth patterns have not been established.

INFLUENCES ON DEVELOPMENTAL TRAJECTORIES OF BRAIN ANATOMY DURING CHILDHOOD AND ADOLESCENCE

Nature/Nurture

One of the fundamental challenges for understanding what factors affect trajectories of brain development is to discern genetic from nongenetic influences. Twin studies are best suited to address these types of questions, and in 2001, we began collaborating with a team of experts in twin research at the Virginia Institute for Psychiatric and Behavioral Genetics and Department of Psychiatry, Virginia Commonwealth University. To date, the sample from the longitudinal study consists of approximately 600 scans from 90 monozygotic (MZ) and 60 dizygotic (DZ) twin pairs.

Structural equation modeling (SEM), which typically uses numeric optimization of a likelihood function to produce parameter values that provide the best fit to the data, is applied to correlation differences between MZ and DZ twins to determine the relative contributions to phenotypic variance of (a) additive genetic, (c) common environmental, or (e) unique environmental factors (Neale and Cardon, 1992). The proportion of variance due to additive genetic effects (also known as "heritability") is high and that due to shared environmental effects is low for most brain morphometric measures (Wallace et al., 2006). Heritability for total cerebrum and lobar volumes (including GM and WM subcompartments) ranged from 0.77–0.88; for the caudate nucleus, it was 0.80, and for the CC heritability was 0.85.

The cerebellum has a distinctive profile, with only 0.49 of variance being due to additive genetic effects (although wide confidence intervals merit cautious interpretation). Pediatric cerebellar development is also noteworthy as being the most sexually dimorphic and among the latest to reach peak volume. These features make the cerebellum a prime target for pediatric neuroimaging studies. Prominent environmental influences on cerebellar development are consistent with its preferential susceptibility to insults such as alcohol, lead, or anoxia. Postnatal neurogenesis of cerebellar

Purkinje cells may also be related to environmental susceptibility (Welsh et al., 2002), although the relationship between this process and volumetric changes remains to be elucidated. Also unclear is whether the unique development and heritability characteristics of the cerebellum are related to its divergence from the other regions soon after neural tube formation; whereas cerebrum, CC, and subcortical structures all are derived from the embryonic prosencephalon, cerebellar tissue is primarily derived from the rhomboencephalon. (Kandel et al., 2000).

Highly heritable brain morphometric measures provide biological markers for inherited traits and may serve as targets for genetic linkage and association studies. These intermediate phenotypes may increase the power to detect quantitative trait loci (QTLs) influencing critical behavioral functions and liability to psychopathology (Gottesman and Gould, 2003). A greater understanding of the forces that guide brain development will help provide a heuristic for developing and implementing more effective interventions in the treatment of brain-based disorders.

Multivariate analyses allow assessment of the degree to which the same genetic or environmental factors contribute to multiple neuroanatomic structures. Like the univariate variables, these interstructure correlations can be parceled into relationships of either genetic or environmental origin. This knowledge is vitally important for interpretation of most of the twin data, including understanding the impact of genes that may affect distributed neural networks and interventions that may have global brain impacts.

Multivariate analyses indicate that shared genetic effects account for more of the variance than structure-specific effects, with a single factor accounting for 60 percent of genetic variability in cortical thickness (Schmitt et al., 2007). After removing effects of global cortical thickness from the thickness of individual gyri, a principal components analysis found that six factors accounted for 58 percent of the variance across 54 cortical regions. A cluster analysis of the same data identified five groups of structures whose members were strongly influenced by the same underlying genetic factors. That most of the genetic variance is determined by genes that are shared between the major gross neural subdivisions is consistent with evolutionary genetic models of brain development that hypothesize global, genetically mediated differences in cell division as the driving force behind interspecies differences in total brain volume (Finlay and Darlington, 1995), as well as with the radial unit hypothesis of neocortical expansion proposed by Rakic (1995).

Comparative neuroanatomic analyses of multiple mammalian species have shown that total brain volume is highly correlated with regional volumes, irrespective of region (including neocortex, striatum, thalamus, and cerebellum), and accounts for the vast majority (> 96%) of the observed volumetric variance in all regions measured except for the olfactory bulb (Fishell, 1997; Darlington et al., 1999). Such strong correlations are thought to reflect a generalized adaptation to specific selective pressures; although it is more expensive, in terms of energy, to expand the computational resources of the entire brain when only specific functions are needed, the molecular adjustments required are far fewer than those required to completely repattern gross neural architecture.

An important aspect of developmental twin studies is assessment of age by heritability interactions. Vulnerabilities of highly heritable neuro-psychiatric illnesses such as anxiety, bipolar disorder, depression, eating disorder, psychosis, and substance abuse are presumably present at birth. However, the peak age for emergence of symptoms in all of these disorders is during adolescence. Age-related changes in heritability may be linked to the timing of gene expression and related to the age of onset of disorders. Knowledge of when certain brain structures are particularly sensitive to genetic or environmental influences during development could also have important educational and/or therapeutic implications. For lobar volumes, WM additive genetic effects account for a greater proportion of the variance with increasing age, whereas for GM, unique environment effects account for a greater proportion of the variance with increasing age (Wallace et al., 2006).

Male/Female

Given that nearly all neuropsychiatric disorders have different prevalence, age of onset, and symptomatology between males and females, sex differences in typical developmental trajectories are highly relevant for studies of pathology. Robust sex differences in developmental trajectories were noted for nearly all structures, with peak volumes generally occurring one to three years earlier for females. Differences in trajectory shapes indicate that male/female differences are not only due to later onset of puberty in boys. The sex differences are also not due solely to body size. Male/female brain size difference remains highly significant when covaried for height and/or weight.

To assess the relative contributions of sex chromosomes and hormones, our group is studying patients with anomalous sex chromosome variations (for example, XXY, XXX, XXXY, XYY) and patients with anomalous hormone levels (for example, congenital adrenal hyperplasia, familial male precocious puberty, Cushing's syndrome).

Specific Genes

As with any quantifiable neuropsychological, clinical, or behavioral feature, people can be categorized into groups based on genotype and the averaged brains of the different genotype groups can be compared statistically. One of the most frequently studied genes in adult populations has been apolipoprotein ε4 (ApoE4). Alleles of the ApoE4 gene modulate risk for Alzheimer's disease, with carriers of the ε4 allele being at increased risk and carriers of ε2 possibly at decreased risk compared with noncarriers. To explore the question of whether ApoE4 alleles have distinct neuroanatomic signatures identifiable in childhood and adolescence, we examined 529 scans from 239 healthy subjects aged 4 to 20 years (Shaw et al., 2007). Although there was no significant association between IQ and genotype, there was a stepwise effect on cortical thickness in the entorhinal and right hippocampal regions, with the ε4 group the thinnest, the ε3 homozygotes in the middle, and the ε2 group the thickest. These data suggest that pediatric assessments might one day be informative for adult onset disorders.

BRAIN-BEHAVIOR CORRELATIONS

As behaviors emanate from the integrated activity of distributed networks, demonstrating straightforward relationships between the size of a given brain structure and a particular behavior or ability has been elusive. Nonetheless, correlations have been identified between some aspects of brain structure and functional capacity. Several studies have shown that there are correlations of brain structural measures with IQ on whole-brain and regional levels (Thompson et al., 2001; Posthuma et al., 2002; Haier et al., 2004; Toga and Thompson, 2004). Relationships between memory function and hippocampal size have also been noted in several species. Food-storing species of birds have larger hippocampi than related non-food-storing species (Krebs et al., 1989; Sherry et al., 1989), whereas in mammals, a similar example can be found in voles. Male voles of the polygamous species travel far and wide in search of mates. They perform better than their female counterparts on laboratory measures of spatial ability and have significantly larger hippocampi (Sherry et al., 1992). Conversely, in the monogamous vole species, which do not show male-female differences in spatial ability, no sexual dimorphism of hippocampal size is seen (Jacobs et al., 1990). In humans also, correlations between memory for stories and left hippocampal volume have also been noted (Lencz et al., 1992; Goldberg et al., 1994). A study of taxi drivers in London found that they had larger hippocampi than controls, thought to be related to their extensive amount of navigational memory required for their work (Maguire et al., 2000).

An important consideration in linking form and function in the brain is that differences in the trajectories of development may in some cases be more informative than the final adult differences. For instance, in our longitudinal study looking at the relationship between cortical thickness and IQ differences in age by cortical thickness, developmental curves were more predictive of IQ than differences in cortical thickness at age twenty years (Shaw et al., 2006).

CONCLUSION

Group differences in anatomical MRI have been reported for nearly all neuropsychiatric disorders. However, because of the large overlap in structure sizes or developmental trajectories, MRI is currently not of diagnostic utility for psychiatric disorders (except to rule out possible central nervous system insults such as tumors, intracranial bleeds, or congenital anomalies as etiologies for the symptoms). There is no identified "lesion" common to all, or even most, children with the most frequently studied disorders of Autism, Attention-Deficit/Hyperactivity Disorder, Childhood-onset Schizophrenia, Dyslexia, Fragile X, Juvenile-onset Bipolar Disorder, Post-Traumatic Stress Disorder, Sydenham's chorea, or Tourette's syndrome.

A more immediately useful aspect of anatomical imaging may be to provide endophenotypes in typical or atypical populations. Endophenotypes are biological markers that can serve as intermediaries between genes and behavior or diagnostic syndromes. Endophenotypes related to a disease may be found in milder form in family members without the full-blown syndrome. Current nonimaging examples in schizophrenia research include eye-tracking abnormalities (Holzman et al., 1974; Calkins and Iacono, 2000) and deficits in P50 suppression (Braff et al., 2001; Braff and Freedman, 2002).

Using brain morphometry as an endophenotype has the potential to create more biologically driven subtypes. This may help to address the important issue of heterogeneity in current polythetic diagnostic schemes such as the *Diagnostic and Statistical Manual of Mental Disorders*, 4th ed., whose diagnostic categories arose from a combination of historical tradition, compatibility with International Classification of Diseases [ICD]-10, clinical and research data, and consensus of the field. More biologically driven subtypes have the potential to be more directly related to specific gene effects.

Remarkable advances in the field of pediatric neuroimaging have opened new windows into our understanding of the living, growing human brain. The mapping of developmental trajectories in typical development lays the groundwork for the next stages of exploring the influences on those trajectories and ultimately using this knowledge to optimize brain development in healthy and clinical populations.

REFERENCES

Allen, L.S., Richey, M.F., Chai, Y.M., and Gorski, R.A. (1991) Sex differences in the corpus callosum of the living human being. *Journal of Neuroscience, 11,* 933–942.

Beaulieu, C., Plewes, C., Paulson, L.A., Roy, D., Snook, L., Concha, L., et al. (2005) Imaging brain connectivity in children with diverse reading ability. *NeuroImage* 25(4), 1266–1271.

Berlucchi, G. (1981) Interhemispheric asymmetries in visual discrimination: a neurophysiological hypothesis. *Doc Ophthalmol Proc Ser, 30,* 87–93.

Braff, D.L., and Freedman, R. (2002) Endophenotypes in studies of the genetics of schizophrenia. In Davis, K.L., Charney, D.S., Coyle, J.T., and Nemeroff, C.B., eds. *Neuropsychopharmacology: The Fifth Generation of Progress.* Philadelphia: Lippincott Williams & Wilkins, pp. 703–716.

Braff, D.L., Geyer, M.A., and Swerdlow, N.R. (2001) Human studies of prepulse inhibition of startle: normal subjects, patient groups, and pharmacological studies. *Psychopharmacology (Berl)* 156(2/3), 234–258.

Brochet, B., and Dousset, V. (1999) Pathological correlates of magnetization transfer imaging abnormalities in animal models and humans with multiple sclerosis. *Neurology, 53*(5 Suppl 3), 7.

Calkins, M.E., and Iacono, W.G. (2000) Eye movement dysfunction in schizophrenia: a heritable characteristic for enhancing phenotype definition. *American Journal of Medical Genetics, 97*(1), 72–76.

Calvert, G.A. (2001) Crossmodal processing in the human brain: insights from functional neuroimaging studies. *Cerebral Cortex, 11*(12), 1110–1123.

Cascio, C.J., Gerig, G., and Piven, J. (2007) Diffusion tensor imaging: application to the study of the developing brain. *Journal of the American Academy of Child and Adolescent Psychiatry, 46*(2), 213–223.

Caviness, V.S.J., Kennedy, D.N., Richelme, C., Rademacher, J., and Filipek, P.A. (1996) The human brain age 7–11 years: a volumetric analysis based on magnetic resonance images. *Cerebral Cortex, 6*(5), 726–736.

Caviness, V.S.J., Lange, N.T., Makris, N., Herbert, M.R., and Kennedy, D.N. (1999) MRI-based brain volumetrics: emergence of a developmental brain science. *Brain & Development, 21*(5), 289–295.

Clark, A.S., MacLusky, N.J., and Goldman-Rakic, P.S. (1988) Androgen binding and metabolism in the cerebral cortex of the developing rhesus monkey. *Endocrinology, 123,* 932–940.

Collins, D.L., Holmes, C.J., Peters, T.M., and Evans, A.C. (1995) Automatic 3-D model-based neuroanatomical segmentation. *Human Brain Mapping, 3,* 190–208.

Cook, N.D. (1986) *The Brain Code. Mechanisms of Information Transfer and the Role of the Corpus Callosum.* London: Methuen.

Cowell, P.E., Allen, L.S., Zalatimo, N.S., and Denenberg, V.H. (1992) A developmental study of sex and age interactions in the human corpus callosum. *Developmental Brain Research, 66,* 187–192.

Darlington, R.B., Dunlop, S.A., and Finlay, B.L. (1999) Neural development in metatherian and eutherian mammals: variation and constraint. *Journal of Comparative Neurolology, 411*(3), 359–368.

Dekaban, A.S. (1977) Tables of cranial and orbital measurements, cranial volume, and derived indexes in males and females from 7 days to 20 years of age. *Annals of Neurology, 2,* 485–491.

Dekaban, A.S., and Sadowsky, D. (1978) Changes in brain weight during the span of human life: relation of brain weights to body heights and body weights. *Annals of Neurology, 4,* 345–356.

Deutsch, G.K., Dougherty, R.F., Bammer, R., Siok, W.T., Gabrieli, J.D., and Wandell, B. (2005) Children's reading performance is correlated with white matter structure measured by diffusion tensor imaging. *Cortex, 41*(3), 354–363.

Diener, E., Sandvik, E., and Larsen, R.F. (1985) Age and sex effects for affect intensity. *Developmental Psychology, 21,* 542–546.

Engelbrecht, V., Rassek, M., Preiss, S., Wald, C., and Modder, U. (1998) Age-dependent changes in magnetization transfer contrast of white matter in the pediatric brain. *American Journal of Neuroradiology, 19*(10), 1923–1929.

Fields, R.D., and Stevens-Graham, B. (2002) New insights into neuron-glia communication. *Science, 298*(5593), 556–562.

Finlay, B.L., and Darlington, R.B. (1995) Linked regularities in the development and evolution of mammalian brains. *Science, 268,* 1578–1584.

Fishell, G. (1997) Regionalization in the mammalian telencephalon. *Current Opinion in Neurobiology, 7*(1), 62–69.

Giedd, J.N., Blumenthal, J., Jeffries, N.O., Castellanos, F.X., Liu, H., Zijdenbos, A., et al. (1999) Brain development during childhood and adolescence: a longitudinal MRI study. *Nature Neuroscience, 2*(10), 861–863.

Giedd, J.N., Blumenthal, J., Jeffries, N.O., Rajapakse, J.C., Vaituzis, A.C., Liu, H., et al. (1999) Development of the human corpus callosum during childhood and adolescence: a longitudinal MRI study. *Progress in NeuroPsychopharmacology and Biological Psychiatry, 23*(4), 571–588.

Giedd, J.N., Castellanos, F.X., Rajapakse, J.C., Kaysen, D., Vaituzis, A.C., Vauss, Y.C., et al. (1995) Cerebral MRI of human brain development – ages 4–18. *Biological Psychiatry, 37*(9), 657.

Giedd, J.N., Shaw, P., Wallace, G.L., Gogtay, N., and Lenroot, R. (2006) Anatomic brain imaging studies of normal and abnormal brain development in children and adolescents. In: Cicchetti, D., ed. *Developmental Psychopathology,* 2nd ed., Vol. 2. Hoboken, NJ: Wiley, pp. 127–196.

Giedd, J.N., Snell, J.W., Lange, N., Rajapakse, J.C., Casey, B.J., Kozuch, P.L., et al. (1996) Quantitative magnetic resonance imaging of human brain development: ages 4–18. *Cerebral Cortex, 6*(4), 551–560.

Giedd, J.N., Vaituzis, A.C., Hamburger, S.D., Lange, N., Rajapakse, J.C., Kaysen, D., et al. (1996) Quantitative MRI of the temporal lobe, amygdala, and hippocampus in normal human development: ages 4–18 years. *Journal of Comparative Neurology, 366*(2), 223–230.

Gogtay, N., Giedd, J.N., Lusk, L., Hayashi, B.S., Greenstein, D., Vaituzis, A.C., et al. (2004) Dynamic mapping of human cortical development during childhood through early adulthood. *Proceedings of the National Academy of Sciences USA, 101*(21), 8174–8179.

Goldberg, T.E., Torrey, E.F., Berman, K.F., and Weinberger, D.R. (1994) Relations between neuropsychological performance and brain morphological and physiological measures in monozygotic twins discordant for schizophrenia. *Psychiatry Research, 55*, 51–61.

Goldstein, J.M., Seidman, L.J., Horton, N.J., Makris, N.K., Kennedy, D.N., Caviness, Jr., V.S., et al. (2001) Normal sexual dimorphism of the adult human brain assessed by in vivo magnetic resonance imaging. *Cerebral Cortex, 11*(6), 490–497.

Gottesman, I., and Gould, T.D. (2003) The endophenotype concept in psychiatry: etymology and strategic intentions. *American Journal of Psychiatry, 160*(4), 636–645.

Haier, R.J., Jung, R.E., Yeo, R.A., Head, K., and Alkire, M.T. (2004) Structural brain variation and general intelligence. *NeuroImage, 23*(1), 425–433.

Holzman, P.S., Proctor, L.R., Levy, D.L., Yasillo, N.J., Meltzer, H.Y., and Hurt, S.W. (1974) Eye-tracking dysfunctions in schizophrenic patients and their relatives. *Archives of General Psychiatry, 31*(2), 143–151.

Huttenlocher, P.R. (1994) Synaptogenesis in human cerebral cortex. In Dawson, G., and Fischer, K., eds. *Human Behavior and the Developing Brain*. New York: Guilford Press, pp. 137–152.

Jacobs, L.F., Gaulin, S.J., Sherry, D.F., and Hoffman, G.E. (1990) Evolution of spatial cognition: sex-specific patterns of spatial behavior predict hippocampal size. *Proceedings of the National Academy of Science USA, 87*, 6349–6352.

Jernigan, T.L., and Tallal, P. (1990) Late childhood changes in brain morphology observable with MRI. *Developmental Medicine and Child Neurology, 32*, 379–385.

Jernigan, T.L., Trauner, D.A., Hesselink, J.R., and Tallal, P.A. (1991) Maturation of human cerebrum observed in vivo during adolescence. *Brain, 114*, 2037–2049.

Jerslid, A.T. (1963) *The Psychology of Adolescence*, 2nd ed. New York: Macmillan.

Kandel, E.R., Schwartz, J.H., and Jessell, T.M. (2000) *Principles of Neural Science*, 4th Ed. New York: McGraw-Hill.

Krebs, J.R., Sherry, D.F., Healy, S.D., Perry, V.H., and Vaccarino, A.L. (1989) Hippocampal specialization of food-storing birds. *Proceedings of the National Academy of Science USA, 86*, 1388–1392.

Lee, K.Y., Kim, T.K., Park, M., Ko, S., Song, I.C., and Cho, I.H. (2004) Age-related changes in conventional and magnetization transfer MR imaging in elderly people: comparison with neurocognitive performance. *Korean Journal of Radiology, 5*(2), 96–101.

Lencz, T., McCarthy, G., Bronen, R.A., Scott, T.M., Inserni, J.A., Sass, K.J., et al. (1992) Quantitative magnetic resonance imaging in temporal lobe epilepsy:

relationship to neuropathology and neuropsychological function. *Annals of Neurology, 31*, 629–637.

Lenroot, R.K., Gogtay, N., Greenstein, D.K., Wells, E.M., Wallace, G.L., Clasen, L.S., et al. (2007) Sexual dimorphism of brain developmental trajectories during childhood and adolescence. *NeuroImage, 36*(4), 1065–1073.

Levy, J. (1985). Interhemispheric collaboration: single mindedness in the asymmetric brain. In: Best, C. T., ed. *Hemisphere Function and Collaboration in the Child*. New York: Academic Press, pp. 11–32.

Liston, C., Watts, R., Tottenham, N., Davidson, M.C., Niogi, S., Ulug, A.M., et al. (2006) Frontostriatal microstructure modulates efficient recruitment of cognitive control. *Cerebral Cortex, 16*(4), 553–560.

Maguire, E.A., Gadian, D.G., Johnsrude, I.S., Good, C.D., Ashburner, J., Frackowiak, R.S., et al. (2000) Navigation-related structural change in the hippocampi of taxi drivers. *Proceedings of the National Academy of Science USA, 97*(8), 4398–4403.

Martin, A., and Chao, L.L. (2001) Semantic memory and the brain: structure and processes. *Current Opinion in Neurobiology 11*(2), 194–201.

Mesulam, M.M. (1998) From sensation to cognition. *Brain, 121*(Pt 6), 1013–1052.

Morse, J.K., Scheff, S.W., and DeKosky, S.T. (1986) Gonadal steroids influence axonal sprouting in the hippocampal dentate gyrus: a sexually dimorphic response. *Exp. Neurology, 94*, 649–658.

Mukherjee, P., and McKinstry, R.C. (2006) Diffusion tensor imaging and tractography of human brain development. *Neuroimaging Clinics of North America, 16*(1), 19–43, vii.

Nagy, Z., Westerberg, H., and Klingberg, T. (2004) Maturation of white matter is associated with the development of cognitive functions during childhood. *J. Cognitive Neuroscience, 16*(7), 1227–1233.

Neale, M.C., and Cardon, L.R. (1992) *Methodology for Genetic Studies of Twins and Families*. Dordrecht: Kluwer Academic.

Niogi, S.N., and McCandliss, B.D. (2006) Left lateralized white matter microstructure accounts for individual differences in reading ability and disability. *Neuropsychologia, 44*(11), 2178–2188.

Nolte, J. (1993) Olfactory and limbic systems. In: Farrell, R., ed. *The Human Brain. An Introduction to its Functional Anatomy*, 3rd Ed. St. Louis: Mosby-Year Book, pp. 397–413.

Pfefferbaum, A., Mathalon, D.H., Sullivan, E.V., Rawles, J.M., Zipursky, R.B., and Lim, K.O. (1994) A quantitative magnetic resonance imaging study of changes in brain morphology from infancy to late adulthood. *Archives of Neurology, 51*(9), 874–887.

Posthuma, D., De Geus, E.J., Baare, W.F., Hulshoff Pol, H.E., Kahn, R.S., and Boomsma, D.I. (2002) The association between brain volume and intelligence is of genetic origin. *Nature Neuroscience, 5*(2), 83–84.

Pujol, J., Vendrell, P., Junque, C., Marti-Vilalta, J.L., and Capdevila, A. (1993) When does human brain development end? Evidence of corpus callosum growth up to adulthood. *Annals of Neurology, 34*, 71–75.

Rakic, P. (1995) A small step for the cell, a giant leap for mankind: a hypothesis of neocortical expansion during evolution. *Trends in Neurosciences, 18*(9), 383–388.

Rauch, R.A., and Jinkins, J.R. (1994) Analysis of cross-sectional area measurements of the corpus callosum adjusted for brain size in male and female subjects from childhood to adulthood. *Behavioural Brain Research*, 64, 65–78.

Reiss, A.L., Abrams, M.T., Singer, H.S., Ross, J.L., and Denckla, M.B. (1996) Brain development, gender and IQ in children. A volumetric imaging study. *Brain*, 119(Pt 5), 1763–17

Rovaris, M., Iannucci, G., Cercignani, M., Sormani, M.P., De Stefano, N., Gerevini, S., et al. (2003) Age-related changes in conventional, magnetization transfer, and diffusion-tensor MR imaging findings: study with whole-brain tissue histogram analysis. *Radiology*, 227(3), 731–738.

Schmithorst, V.J., Wilke, M., Dardzinski, B.J., and Holland, S.K. (2005) Cognitive functions correlate with white matter architecture in a normal pediatric population: a diffusion tensor MRI study. *Human Brain Mapping*, 26(2), 139–147.

Schmitt, J.E., Lenroot, R.K., Wallace, G.L., Ordaz, S., Taylor, K.N., Kabani N., et al. (2008) Identification of genetically mediated cortical networks: a multivariate study of pediatric twins and siblings. *Cerebral Cortex*, 18(8), 1737–1747.

Shanks, M.F., Rockel, A.J., and Powel, T.P.S. (1975) The commissural fiber connections of the primary somatic sensory cortex. *Brain Research*, 98, 166–171.

Shaw, P., Greenstein, D., Lerch, J., Clasen, L., Lenroot, R., Gogtay, N., et al. (2006) Intellectual ability and cortical development in children and adolescents. *Nature*, 440(7084), 676–679.

Shaw, P., Lerch, J.P., Pruessner, J.C., Taylor, K.N., Rose, A.B., Greenstein, D., et al. (2007) Cortical morphology in children and adolescents with different apolipoprotein E gene polymorphisms: an observational study. *Lancet Neurology*, 6(6), 494–500.

Sherry, D.F., Jacobs, L.F., and Gaulin, S.J. (1992) Spatial memory and adaptive specialization of the hippocampus [see comments]. *Trends in Neurosciences*, 15, 298–303.

Sherry, D.F., Vaccarino, A.L., Buckenham, K., and Herz, R.S. (1989) The hippocampal complex of food-storing birds. *Brain, Behavior and Evolution*, 34, 308–317.

Sowell, E.R., and Jernigan, T.L. (1998) Further MRI evidence of late brain maturation: Limbic volume increases and changing asymmetries during childhood and adolescence. *Developmental Neuropsychology*, 14(4), 599–617.

Sowell, E.R., Peterson, B.S., Thompson, P.M., Welcome, S.E., Henkenius, A.L., and Toga, A.W. (2003) Mapping cortical change across the human life span. *Nature Neuroscience*, 6(3), 309–315.

Sowell, E.R., Thompson, P.M., Holmes, C.J., Batth, R., Jernigan, T.L., and Toga, A.W. (1999) Localizing age-related changes in brain structure between childhood and adolescence using statistical parametric mapping. *NeuroImage*, 9(6 Pt 1), 587–597.

Sowell, E.R., Thompson, P.M., Holmes, C.J., Jernigan, T.L., and Toga, A.W. (1999) In vivo evidence for post-adolescent brain maturation in frontal and striatal regions. *Nature Neuroscience*, 2(10), 859–861.

Sowell, E.R., Thompson, P.M., Tessner, K.D., and Toga, A.W. (2001) Mapping continued brain growth and gray matter density reduction in dorsal frontal cortex: inverse relationships during post-adolescent brain maturation. *Journal of Neuroscience*, 21(22), 8819–8829.

Suzuki, Y., Matsuzawa, H., Kwee, I.L., and Nakada, T. (2003) Absolute eigenvalue diffusion tensor analysis for human brain maturation. *NMR in Biomedicine*, *16*(5), 257–260.

Thompson, P.M., Cannon, T.D., Narr, K.L., van Erp, T., Poutanen, V.P., Huttunen, M., et al. (2001) Genetic influences on brain structure. *Nature Neuroscience*, *4*(12), 1253–1258.

Thompson, P.M., Giedd, J.N., Woods, R.P., MacDonald, D., Evans, A.C., and Toga, A.W. (2000) Growth patterns in the developing brain detected by using continuum mechanical tensor maps. *Nature*, *404*(6774), 190–193.

Thompson, P.M., Hayashi, K.M., Sowell, E.R., Gogtay, N., Giedd, J.N., Rapoport, J.L., et al. (2004) Mapping cortical change in Alzheimer's disease, brain development, and schizophrenia. *NeuroImage*, *23*(Suppl 1), S2–S18.

Toga, A.W., and Thompson, P.M. (2005) Genetics of brain structure and intelligence. *Annual Review of Neuroscience*, *28*, 1–23.

van Buchem, M.A., Steens, S.C., Vrooman, H.A., Zwinderman, A.H., McGowan, J.C., Rassek, M., et al. (2001) Global estimation of myelination in the developing brain on the basis of magnetization transfer imaging: a preliminary study. *American Journal of Neuroradiology*, *22*(4), 762–766.

Wallace, G.L., Schmitt, J.E., Lenroot, R.K., Viding, E., Ordaz, S., Rosenthal, M.A., et al. (2006) A pediatric twin study of brain morphometry. *Journal of Child Psychology and Psychiatry*, *47*(10), 987–993.

Wechsler, D. (1974) *Wechsler Intelligence Scale for Children – Revised*. New York: The Psychological Corporation.

Welsh, J.P., Yuen, G., Placantonakis, D.G., Vu, T.Q., Haiss, F., O'Hearn, E., et al. (2002) Why do Purkinje cells die so easily after global brain ischemia? Aldolase C, EAAT4, and the cerebellar contribution to posthypoxic myoclonus. *Advances in Neurology*, *89*, 331–359.

Whitford, T.J, Rennie, C.J., Grieve, S.M, Clark, C.R., Gordon, E. E., and Williams, L. M. (2007) Brain maturation in adolescence: concurrent changes in neuroanatomy and neurophysiology. *Human Brain Mapping*, *28*(3), 228–237.

Zaidel, D., and Sperry, R. W. (1974) Memory impairment after commissurotomy in man. *Brain*, *97*, 263–272.

3

Adolescent Risk Taking: A Social Neuroscience Perspective

LAURENCE STEINBERG

Temple University

It is widely agreed among experts in the study of adolescent health and development that the greatest threats to the well-being of young people in industrialized societies come from preventable and often self-inflicted causes, including automobile and other accidents (which together account for nearly half of all fatalities among U.S. youth), violence, drug and alcohol use, and sexual risk taking (Ozer & Irwin, 2009). Although considerable progress has been made in the prevention and treatment of disease and chronic illness among this age group, similar gains have not been made with respect to reducing the morbidity and mortality that result from risky and reckless behavior (Hein, 1988). Whereas rates of certain types of adolescent risk taking, such as driving under the influence of alcohol or having unprotected sex, have dropped over time, the prevalence of risky behavior among teenagers remains high, and there has been no decline in adolescents' risk behavior in several years (Centers for Disease Control and Prevention, 2006).

It is also noteworthy that adolescents engage in more risky behavior than adults, although the magnitude of age differences in risk taking varies as a function of the specific risk in question and the age of the "adolescents" and "adults" used as comparison groups; rates of risk taking are high among eighteen- to twenty-one-year-olds, for instance, some of whom may be classified as adolescents and some who may be classified as adults. Nonetheless, as a general rule, adolescents and young adults are more likely than adults older than twenty-five to binge-drink, smoke cigarettes, have casual sex partners, engage in violent and other criminal behavior, and have fatal or serious automobile accidents, the majority of which are caused by reckless driving or driving under the influence of alcohol. Because many forms of risk behavior initiated in adolescence elevate the risk for the behavior in adulthood (e.g., drug use), and because some forms of risk taking by adolescents put individuals of other ages at risk (e.g., reckless driving, criminal behavior), public health experts agree that reducing the rate of risk taking by young people would make a substantial improvement in the overall well-being of the population (Steinberg, 2004).

The primary approach to reducing adolescent risk taking has been through educational programs, most of them school-based, but there is reason to be highly skeptical about the effectiveness of this approach. According to the AddHealth survey (Bearman, Jones, & Udry, 1997), virtually all American adolescents have received some form of educational intervention designed to reduce smoking, drinking, drug use, and unprotected sex. Nevertheless, data from the Youth Risk Behavior Survey, conducted by the Centers for Disease Control and Prevention, indicate that more than one-third of high school students did not use a condom either the first time or even the last time they had sexual intercourse, and that during the year prior to the survey, nearly 30 percent of adolescents rode in a car driven by someone who had been drinking, more than 25 percent reported multiple episodes of binge-drinking, and nearly 25 percent were regular cigarette smokers (Centers for Disease Control and Prevention, 2006).

It is true, naturally, that the situation might be even worse were it not for these educational efforts. But most systematic research on health education indicates that even the best programs are far more successful at changing individuals' knowledge than in altering their behavior (Steinberg 2008). Indeed, in the United States, significantly more than a billion dollars are spent each year educating adolescents about the dangers of smoking, drinking, drug use, unprotected sex, and reckless driving – all with surprisingly little impact. Most taxpayers would be surprised – perhaps shocked – to learn that vast expenditures of public dollars are invested in health, sex, and driver education programs that either do not work, such as D.A.R.E. (Ennett, Tobler, Ringwall, & Flewelling, 1994), abstinence education (Trenholm, Devaney, Fortson, Quay, Wheeler, & Clark, 2007), or driver training (National Research Council, 2007), or are, at best, of unproven or unstudied effectiveness (Steinberg, 2007).

The high rate of risky behavior among adolescents relative to adults, despite massive, ongoing, and costly efforts to educate teenagers about its potentially harmful consequences, has been the focus of much theorizing and empirical research by developmental scientists for at least twenty-five years. Most of this work has been informative, but in an unexpected way. In general, where investigators have looked to find differences between adolescents and adults that would explain the more frequent risky behavior of youth, they have not been successful. Among the widely held beliefs about adolescent risk taking that have *not* been supported empirically are that adolescents are irrational or deficient in their information processing, or that they reason about risk in fundamentally different ways than adults, that adolescents do not perceive risks where adults do, or are more likely to believe that they are invulnerable, and that adolescents are less risk-averse than adults (see Albert & Steinberg, 2011, for a review). None of these assertions is correct: The logical reasoning and basic information-processing abilities of sixteen-year-olds are comparable to those of adults; adolescents are no worse than adults at perceiving risk or estimating their vulnerability to it (and, like adults, *over*estimate the dangerousness associated with various risky behaviors); and increasing the salience of the risks associated with making a poor or potentially dangerous decision has comparable effects on adolescents and adults (Millstein & Halpern-Felsher, 2002; Reyna & Farley, 2006; Rivers, Reyna, & Mills, 2008; Steinberg & Cauffman, 1996). Indeed, most studies find few, if any, age differences in individuals' evaluations of the risks inherent in a wide range of dangerous behaviors (e.g., driving while drunk, having unprotected sex), in their judgments about the seriousness of the consequences that might result from risky behavior, or in the ways that they evaluate the relative costs and benefits of these activities (Beyth-Marom et al., 1993). In sum, adolescents' greater involvement than adults in risk taking does not stem from ignorance, irrationality, delusions of invulnerability, or faulty calculations (Reyna & Farley, 2006).

The fact that adolescents are as knowledgeable, logical, reality-based, and accurate in the ways in which they think about risky activity as their elders, but nevertheless engage in higher rates of risky behavior, raises important considerations for both scientists and practitioners. For the former, this observation pushes us to think differently about the factors that may contribute to age differences in risky behavior and to ask what it is that changes between adolescence and adulthood that might account for these differences. For the latter, it helps explain why educational interventions have been so limited in their success, suggests that providing adolescents with information and decision-making skills may be a misguided strategy, and argues that we need a new approach to public health interventions aimed at reducing adolescent risk-taking if it is adolescents' actual behavior that we wish to change. In this chapter, I propose an approach to the problem that is grounded in developmental neuroscience.

The last decade has been one of enormous and sustained interest in patterns of brain development during adolescence and young adulthood. Enabled by the growing accessibility and declining cost of structural and functional magnetic resonance imaging (MRI) and other imaging techniques, such as diffusion tensor imaging (DTI), an expanding network of scientists have begun to map out the course of changes in brain structure between childhood and adulthood, describe age differences in brain activity during this period of development, and, to a more modest degree, link findings on the changing morphology and functioning of the brain to age differences in behavior (for a recent review, see Paus, 2009). Although it is wise to heed the cautions of those who have raised concerns about "brain overclaim" (Morse, 2006), there is no doubt that our understanding of the neural underpinnings of adolescent psychological development is shaping – and reshaping – the ways in which developmental scientists think about normative (Steinberg, 2009) and atypical (Steinberg, Dahl, Keating, Kupfer, Masten, & Pine, 2006) development in adolescence.

In this chapter, I present findings from a program of behavioral research that is informed by the study of adolescent brain development. Before proceeding, it is important to acknowledge that our knowledge of changes in brain structure and function during adolescence far exceeds our understanding of the actual links between these neurobiological changes and adolescent behavior (Steinberg, 2010). Frequently, contemporaneous processes of adolescent neural and behavioral development – for example, the synaptic pruning that occurs in the prefrontal cortex during adolescence and improvements in long-term planning – are presented as causally linked without data that even correlates these developments, much less demonstrates that the former (brain) influences the latter (behavior), rather than the reverse. Indeed, in light of evidence of considerable brain plasticity in adolescence, it is likely that brain development in adolescence is a product of both maturation and experience. It is therefore wise to be cautious about simple accounts of adolescent behavior that attribute changes in these phenomena directly to changes in brain structure or function.

It is important to be especially cautious about making sweeping claims about age differences in risky behavior from neuroscientific studies, because individuals are more likely to view the results of behavioral research as credible when a neuroscience narrative is attached to the social science account (Steinberg, 2009). In one widely cited study, when presented with sensible accounts of psychological phenomena, subjects were equally satisfied regardless of whether the explanations referred to the brain. But when presented with circular or otherwise logically suspect accounts, subjects were dissatisfied when the explanations did not contain information about the brain but satisfied when they did (Weisberg et al., 2008).

These cautions notwithstanding, the current state of our knowledge about adolescent brain development and possible brain-behavior links during this period, although incomplete, is nonetheless sufficient to offer some insight into the study of adolescent risk taking. Two fundamental questions about the development of risk taking in adolescence have motivated the program of work described in this chapter. First, why does risk taking increase between childhood and adolescence? Second, why does risk taking decline between adolescence and adulthood? As I hope to demonstrate, developmental neuroscience provides clues that may lead us toward an answer to both questions.

A DUAL-SYSTEMS MODEL OF ADOLESCENT RISK TAKING

In the past several years, a new perspective on risk taking and decision making during adolescence has emerged that is informed by advances in developmental neuroscience (Casey, Getz, & Galvan 2008; Steinberg 2008). According to this view, risky behavior in adolescence is the product of the interaction between changes in two distinct neurobiological systems: a "socioemotional" system, which is localized in limbic and paralimbic areas of the brain, including the amygdala, ventral striatum, orbitofrontal cortex, medial prefrontal cortex, and superior temporal sulcus; and a "cognitive control" system, which is mainly composed of the lateral prefrontal and parietal cortices and those parts of the anterior cingulate cortex to which they are interconnected (Steinberg, 2008). According to this dual-systems model, adolescent risk taking is hypothesized to be stimulated by a rapid and dramatic increase in dopaminergic activity within the socioemotional system around the time of puberty, which is presumed to lead to increases in reward seeking. However, this increase in reward seeking precedes the structural maturation of the cognitive control system and its connections to areas of the socioemotional system, a maturational process that is gradual, unfolds over the course of adolescence, and permits more advanced self-regulation and impulse control. The temporal gap between the arousal of the socioemotional system, which is an early adolescent development, and the full maturation of the cognitive control system, which occurs later, creates a period of heightened vulnerability to risk taking during middle adolescence (Steinberg, 2008).

Neurobiological evidence in support of the dual-systems model is impressive. A growing literature, derived primarily from rodent studies but with implications for human development, indicates that the remodeling of the dopaminergic system within the socioemotional network involves an initial postnatal rise and then, starting in preadolescence, a subsequent reduction of dopamine receptor density in the striatum and prefrontal cortex. This pattern is more pronounced among males than females (Sisk & Foster, 2004; Teicher, Andersen, & Hostetter, Jr., 1995). As a result of this remodeling, dopaminergic activity in the prefrontal cortex increases significantly in early adolescence and is higher during this period than before or after. Because dopamine plays a critical role in the brain's reward circuitry, the increase, reduction, and redistribution of dopamine receptor concentration around puberty, especially in projections from the limbic system to the prefrontal area, is likely to increase reward-seeking behavior.

There is equally compelling neurobiological evidence for changes in brain structure and function during adolescence and early adulthood that facilitate improvements in self-regulation and permit individuals to modulate their inclinations to seek rewards, although this development is presumed to unfold along a different timetable and be independent of puberty (Paus, 2009). As a consequence of synaptic pruning and the continued myelination of prefrontal brain regions, there are improvements over the course of adolescence in many aspects of executive function, such as response inhibition, ahead-of-time planning, risks and rewards evaluation, and the simultaneous consideration of multiple sources of information. There is also improved coordination of affect and cognition, which is facilitated by the increased connectivity between regions associated with the socioemotional and cognitive control systems (Steinberg, 2010).

Research on adolescent behavioral development has not kept pace with advances in our understanding of brain development, however, and the notion that the developmental course of reward seeking (thought to increase mainly between preadolescence and middle adolescence) differs from that of impulse control (thought to increase gradually over adolescence and early adulthood) has not been examined systematically. Thus, although there is good evidence that risk taking is higher during adolescence than during preadolescence or adulthood (as evidenced by age differences in a wide range of risky activity, including criminal behavior, reckless driving, unprotected sex, and binge-drinking; Steinberg 2008), it is not clear whether the increase and then decline in risk taking that occurs at this time is due to changes in reward seeking, changes in impulse control, or some combination of the two. At least one recent study (Galvan, Hare, Voss, Glover, & Casey, 2007) indicates that individuals' self-reported likelihood of engaging in risky behavior is more strongly connected to reward processing than to impulsivity, but studies of this issue are sparse. To examine whether reward seeking and impulsivity develop along different timetables, it is necessary to have conceptually and empirically distinct measures of each.

Dahl (2004) has described reward seeking as one of a suite of developmental domains that appear to be linked to puberty-specific maturational changes. Consistent with this, animal studies indicate that increases in reward seeking are coincident with pubertal maturation, although it is not clear whether these increases are caused by increases in pubertal hormones or merely coincident with them (Sisk & Foster, 2004; Spear 2000). It is plausible that changes in brain systems that subserve reward seeking are biologically "programmed" to occur simultaneously with reproductive maturation, to encourage the sort of risk taking that would be evolutionarily adaptive (Casey et al., 2008; Steinberg, 2008). Research linking reward seeking to pubertal maturation among humans is scarce, but at least one study has shown that sensation seeking and pubertal maturation are positively correlated (Martin et al., 2001). Sensation seeking (which is highly related to reward seeking) also is positively correlated with levels of testosterone and estradiol among both males and females of college age (Zuckerman, Buchsbaum, & Murphy, 1980). Regardless of whether sensation seeking (or reward seeking) is directly or indirectly associated with pubertal maturation, however, there is clear support for the prediction that this behavior increases during the first part of adolescence.

Self-report studies of age differences in impulsivity that span adolescence and adulthood are even rarer than those examining reward seeking. Galvan and colleagues (2007) report a significant negative correlation between chronological age and impulsivity (using the Connors Impulsivity Scale) in a sample of individuals ranging in age from seven to twenty-nine years, suggesting that impulse control continues to develop over the course of adolescence and early adulthood. Leshem and Glicksohn (2007) likewise report a significant decline in impulsivity from ages fourteen-to-sixteen to twenty-to-twenty-two on both the Eysenk and Barratt impulsiveness scales. Another study found higher scores on the Barratt Impulsiveness Scale for high school, relative to college, students, although the authors attribute the finding to a filtering effect, whereby highly impulsive and presumably low-achieving high school students do not continue on to college (Stanford, Greve, Boudreaux, Mathias, & Brumbelow, 1996). Although these studies all suggest a steady decline in impulsivity from childhood through adolescence and into adulthood, there is a clear need for normative data from a large sample across a broad age range.

The present chapter summarizes results from a program of research my colleagues and I have recently completed, designed to examine age differences in reward seeking and cognitive control between the ages of ten and thirty (for more detailed presentations of the results discussed in this chapter, see Cauffman et al., 2010; Steinberg et al., 2008; Steinberg et al., 2009). Our study breaks new ground in several respects. First, it is the first study of these phenomena to span a wide enough age range to examine the developmental course of each phenomenon from preadolescence through early adulthood. We studied participants as young as ten because we were interested in examining the relationship between reward seeking and pubertal maturation and thus needed to include some participants who were prepubertal or in the early stages of puberty. On the other hand, we included participants as old as thirty because of recent neurobiological studies indicating that brain regions important for self-regulation may not be fully mature until the mid-twenties.

Second, we made a concerted effort to measure self-control and reward seeking independently within the sample. Many measures of these constructs conflate them; for example, inspection of the Zuckerman Sensation Seeking Scale, the most widely used self-report measure of this construct, reveals that many items explicitly measure impulsivity (e.g., "I often do things on impulse"). However, if these phenomena develop along different timetables and are subserved by different brain systems, it is essential to have separate measures of them. In fact, we hypothesize that reward seeking is curvilinearly related to chronological age, increasing during early adolescence (coincident with pubertal maturation) but declining or remaining stable thereafter, whereas impulsivity declines gradually over this same age period.

Finally, we employed both self-report and performance measures of key constructs. For the most part, developmental studies of impulsivity and reward seeking have relied on self-reports. Although these measures are useful for gauging self-perceptions (which may in fact be accurate), it is important to have behavioral assessments as well. In view of widely held stereotypes of teenagers as deficient in self-control and highly oriented toward novelty seeking, it would not be surprising to find that adolescents describe themselves this way. Whether they actually behave this way, of course, is a different question.

THE STUDY

Our study employed five data-collection sites: Denver, Irvine (California), Los Angeles, Philadelphia, and Washington, D.C. Participants were recruited via newspaper advertisements and flyers posted at community organizations, Boys and Girls clubs, churches, community colleges, and local places of business in neighborhoods targeted to have an average household education level of "some college" according to 2000 U.S. Census data. Individuals who were interested in the study were asked to call the research office listed on the flyer. Members of the research team described the nature of the study to the participant over the telephone and invited those interested to participate.

The sample included 935 individuals between the ages of 10 and 30 years, recruited to yield an age distribution designed both to facilitate the examination of age differences within the adolescent decade and to compare adolescents of different ages with young adults. To have cells with sufficiently large and comparably sized subsamples for purposes of data analysis, age groups were created as follows: 10–11 years ($N = 116$), 12–13 years ($N = 137$), 14–15 years ($N = 128$), 16–17 years ($N = 141$), 18–21 years ($N = 138$), 22–25 years ($N = 136$), and 26–30 years ($N = 123$).

Participants reported their age, gender, ethnicity, and household education. Individuals younger than eighteen reported their parents' education, whereas participants eighteen and older reported their own educational attainment (used as a proxy for socioeconomic status [SES]). Participants were predominantly working and middle class. The age groups did not differ with respect to gender or ethnicity but did differ (modestly) with respect to SES. As such, all subsequent analyses controlled for this variable. The sample was evenly split between males (49 percent) and females (51 percent) and was ethnically diverse, with 30 percent African-American, 15 percent Asian, 21 percent Latino(a), 24 percent White, and 10 percent other.

Data collection took place either at one of the participating university's offices or at a location in the community where it was possible to administer the test battery in a quiet and private location. Before beginning, participants were provided verbal and written explanations of the study, their confidentiality was assured, and their written consent or assent was obtained. For participants who were younger than eighteen, informed consent was obtained from either a parent or guardian.

Participants completed a two-hour assessment that consisted of a series of computerized tasks, a set of computer-administered self-report measures, a demographic questionnaire, several computerized tests of general intellectual function (e.g., digit span, working memory), and an assessment of intelligence quotient (IQ). Because performance on measures of reward seeking and impulse control is correlated with intelligence, we administered the *Wechsler Abbreviated Scale of Intelligence* (WASI) Full-Scale IQ Two-Subtest (FSIQ-2) (Psychological Corporation, 1999) to produce an estimate of general intellectual ability based on two (Vocabulary and Matrix Reasoning) out of the four subtests. The WASI can be administered in approximately fifteen minutes and is correlated with the Wechsler Intelligence Scale for Children ($r = .81$) and the Wechsler Adult Intelligence Scale ($r = .87$). There were small but significant differences between the age groups in IQ, and, accordingly, this variable was controlled in all subsequent analyses.

The tasks were administered in individual interviews. Research assistants were present to monitor the participant's progress, reading aloud the instructions as each new task was presented and providing assistance as needed. To keep participants engaged in the assessment, participants were told that they would receive $35 for participating in the study and that they could obtain up to a total of $50 (or, for the participants younger than fourteen, an additional prize of approximately $15 in value) based on their performance on the video tasks. In actuality, we paid all participants ages fourteen to thirty the full $50, and all participants ages ten to thirteen received $35 plus the prize. This strategy was used to increase the motivation to perform well on the tasks but ensure that no participants were penalized for their performance. All procedures were approved by the institutional review board (IRB) of the university associated with each data-collection site.

In this chapter, I report on age differences in self-report measures of impulsivity and reward seeking, and in performance on a computerized version of the Tower of London task (used as a behavioral measure of impulsivity), a computerized adaptation of the Iowa Gambling Task (IGT) (used as a behavioral measure of reward seeking), and a computerized version of a Delay Discounting task (used as a behavioral measure of preference for immediate versus delayed rewards).

Self-Reported Impulsivity

A widely used self-report measure of impulsivity, the Barratt Impulsiveness Scale, Version 11 (Patton, Stanford, & Barratt, 1995), was part of the questionnaire battery; the measure has been shown to have good construct, convergent, and discriminant validity. Based on inspection of the full list of items (the scale has six subscales comprising thirty-four items) and some exploratory factor analyses, we opted to use only eighteen items ($\alpha = .73$) from three six-item subscales: motor impulsivity (e.g., "I act on the spur of the moment"), inability to delay gratification (e.g., "I spend more money than I should"), and lack of perseverance (e.g., "It's hard for me to think about two different things at the same time"). Each item is scored on a four-point scale

(Rarely/Never, Occasionally, Often, Almost Always/Always), with higher scores indicative of greater impulsivity. Subscales were averaged to form a total impulsivity score. Although our composite only includes three of the six subscales, the correlation between our measure and one that includes items from all six subscales is .87. The eighteen-item scale showed excellent fit to the data (NFI = .912, CFI = .952, RMSEA = .033), and reliability of the scale is α = .73.

Self-Reported Reward Seeking

Self-reported reward seeking was assessed using a subset of six items from the Sensation Seeking Scale (Zuckerman, Eysenck, & Eysenck, 1978). As I noted earlier, many of the items on the full nineteen-item Zuckerman scale appear to measure impulsivity, not sensation seeking. In view of our interest in distinguishing between impulsivity and reward seeking, we used only the six Zuckerman items that clearly index reward or novelty seeking (e.g., "I like to have new and exciting experiences and sensations even if they are a little frightening"; "I'll try anything once"; "I sometimes do 'crazy' things just for fun"). All items were answered as either True (coded 1) or False (coded 0), and item scores were averaged. The resulting six-item scale showed an excellent fit to the data (NFI = .955, CFI = .967, RMSEA = .053) and good internal consistency (α = .70).

Tower of London

This task, which is typically used to measure planning and executive function, was used to generate a behavioral index of impulsivity. In the version of the task employed in the present study (Berg & Byrd, 2002), the subject is presented with pictures of two sets of three colored balls distributed across three rods, one of which can hold three balls, one two balls, and the last only one ball. The first picture shows the starting positioning of the three balls, and the second depicts the goal position. The subject is asked to move the balls in the starting arrangement to match the other arrangement in as few moves as necessary, using the computer cursor to "drag" and "drop" each ball. Five sets of four problems are presented, beginning with four that can be solved in three moves and progressing to those that require a minimum of seven moves. In the administration of the task, the starting and goal positions are displayed, and the subject takes as much (or as little) time as necessary before making each move. Hasty performance, particularly with respect to first moves on each problem, has been linked to response inhibition difficulties among children, adolescents, and adults (Asato, Sweeney, & Luna, 2006). Thus, in the current study, shorter latencies to first move indicate greater impulsivity.

Modified IGT

In the version of the task employed here, individuals attempt to earn pretend money by playing or passing cards from from different decks presented on the computer screen. As in the original task (Bechara, Damasio, Damasio, & Anderson, 1994), two of the decks are advantageous and result in a monetary gain over repeated play; the other two decks are disadvantageous and produce a net loss. The task was modified such that participants made a play/pass decision with regard to one of four decks preselected on each trial, rather than deciding to choose to draw from any of four decks on any trial, as in the original task. This type of modification permits one to independently track behavior that reflects reward seeking (i.e., selecting advantageous decks) versus behavior that reflects cost aversion (i.e., avoiding disadvantageous decks) (Peters & Slovic, 2000). In addition to modifying the response option (i.e., play/pass), we also modified the outcome feedback, such that participants received information on the net gain or loss associated with a card rather than information on both a gain and the loss separately (Bechara et al., 1994). This modification was made to equate working memory loads across age groups during feedback and also to ensure that participants did not unequally weight the rewards and punishments within a given trial. The task was administered in three blocks of forty trials each.

Delay Discounting

The delay discounting paradigm is widely used by behavioral economists and social and clinical psychologists in the assessment of individuals' preference for future versus immediate outcomes, but surprisingly few studies have examined age differences in delay discounting (see Steinberg et al., 2009, for a summary). In this paradigm, the respondent is asked to choose between an immediate reward of less value (e.g., $400 today) and a variety of delayed rewards of more value (e.g., $1,000 a year from now?), and the outcome of interest is the extent to which respondents prefer the delayed and more valuable reward over the immediately available but less valuable one. In our adaptation of the task, the amount of the delayed reward was held constant at $1,000. We varied the time to delay in six blocks (one day, one week, one month, three months, six months, and one year), presented in a random order. For each block, the starting value of the immediate reward was $200, $500, or $800, randomly determined for each participant. The respondent was then asked to choose between an immediate reward of a given amount and a delayed reward of $1,000. If the immediate reward was preferred, the subsequent question presented an immediate reward midway between the prior one and zero (i.e., a lower figure). If the delayed reward was preferred, the subsequent question presented an immediate reward midway between the prior one and $1,000 (i.e., a higher figure). Participants then worked their way through a total of nine ascending and descending choices until their responses converged and their preference for the immediate and delayed reward were equal, at a value reflecting the "discounted" value of the delayed reward (i.e., the subjective value of the delayed reward if it were offered immediately; Green, Myerson, & Macaux, 2005), referred to as the "indifference point" (Ohmura, Takahashi, Kitamura, & Wehr, 2006). For each individual, we computed the indifference point for each delay interval as well as the average indifference point. An individual with a relatively lower indifference point is relatively more drawn to the prospect of an immediate reward.

FINDINGS

The organizing hypothesis guiding our work is that reward seeking increases in early adolescence and then declines, but that impulsivity gradually declines with age, continuing through late adolescence and into young adulthood. As a consequence of these different patterns of development, middle adolescence (ages fourteen to seventeen) is expected to be a period of heightened risk taking, during which individuals are especially inclined to seek rewards (which leads to higher levels of sensation seeking) but are not yet able to regulate their behavior in a way that balances the allure of potential rewards with the risk of potential costs. As I noted earlier in the chapter, many forms of risk taking follow this general pattern, and although the specific chronological age at which risky behavior peaks varies from one domain of behavior to the next (e.g., crime peaks around age seventeen whereas binge-drinking peaks in the early twenties), risky behavior generally increases over the course of adolescence and then declines during young adulthood. My suspicion is that differences in peak ages likely reflect differential opportunity to engage in the specific risk behavior in question (i.e., the peak in crime occurs before the peak in binge-drinking because the sale of alcohol is restricted to individuals older than twenty-one, whereas

engaging in crime is an "equal opportunity" risk behavior) and not differences in neurobiological or psychological development.

We examined age differences in self-reports of impulsivity and reward
seeking via two sets of hierarchical multiple regression analyses. Age, IQ,
and socioeconomic status (SES) were entered on the first step (to test for
the linear relationship between age and the outcome of interest, while
controlling for the small age group differences in IQ and SES), and the
quadratic term for age was entered on the second step (to test for the curvilinear relation between age and the outcome of interest). As predicted,
we found significant linear and curvilinear effects of age on reward seeking ($ß = -.115$, $p < .001$, and $ß = -.437$, $p < .005$, for the linear and quadratic
terms, respectively) but only a linear effect of age on impulsivity ($ß = -.149$,
$p < .001$, and $ß = -.091$, ns, respectively). Figure 3.1 illustrates these two age
patterns. Consistent with our hypothesis, reward seeking increases during
the first half of adolescence and then declines steadily from age sixteen on.
In contrast, impulsivity declines or remains stable over the entire twenty-
year period studied.

These age differences in self-characterizations are evident in performance on the behavioral tasks designed to measure these same constructs. Participants' time before making their first move on the Tower
of London task was our chief behavioral index of impulse control. Age
differences on this measure were examined using a repeated-measures
analysis of covariance (ANCOVA), with age, gender, and ethnicity as the
independent variables; IQ and SES as covariates; and individuals' average time (in milliseconds) before making a first move at each level of
problem difficulty (three, four, five, six, and seven moves) as a five-level
within-subjects factor. We found a significant effect of age on average time
to first move, with older subjects taking more time before moving than
younger ones ($F(6,813) = 17.58$, $p < .001$). More interestingly, however, and as
Figure 3.2 illustrates, there is a significant interaction between age and
problem difficulty, such that with increasing problem difficulty, older, but
not younger, subjects wait longer before their first move ($F(24,3252) = 8.976$,
$p < .001$). Indeed, the three youngest groups generally do not wait any longer
before their first move in the most difficult (seven-move) problems than in
the easiest ones (three moves).

Because Tower of London performance is influenced by working memory as well as inhibitory control (Asato et al., 2006), and because there are
gains in working memory during the first part of adolescence (Keating,
2004), it was important to ensure that the observed age differences in time
to first move were not simply due to age differences in working memory.

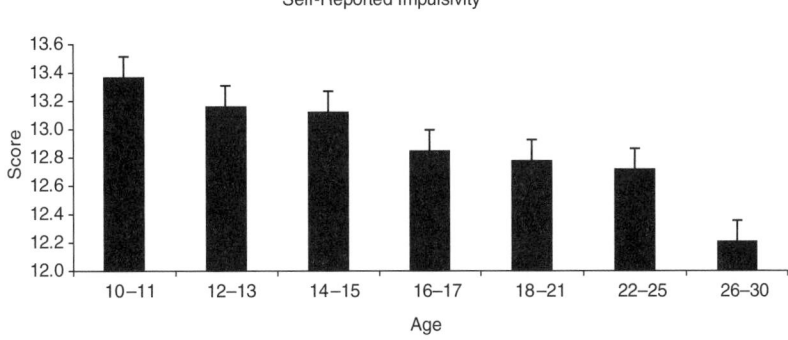

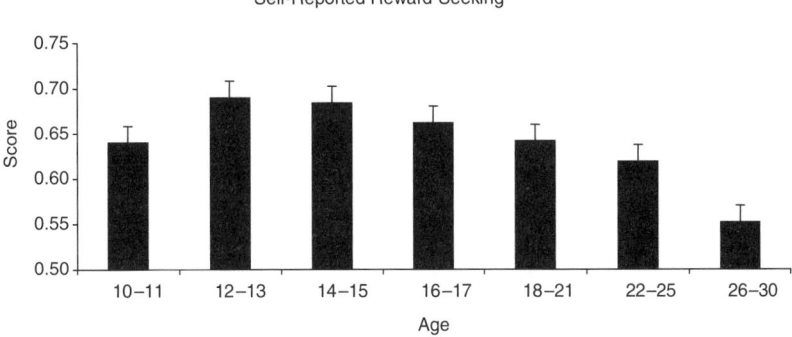

FIGURE 3.1. Age differences in self-reported impulsivity and reward seeking.
Note: Impulsivity scores can range from 6 to 24. Reward-seeking scores can range
from 0 to 1. The linear trend for impulsivity is significant at $p < .001$; the curvilinear trend is not significant. The linear and quadratic trends for reward seeking are
significant at $p < .001$ and $p < .005$, respectively (Steinberg et al., 2008).

The test battery included a test of resistance to interference in working
memory (Thompson-Schill, 2002). In this task, participants saw four probe
letters on the screen, followed by a screen displaying a target letter. They
were then asked whether the target was among the four probes. An overall
accuracy of working memory score was computed by averaging the number of correct responses across all experimental trials. When we repeated
our analyses of age differences in time to first move, controlling for age
differences in working memory, the results were unchanged. In more
recent analyses of these data looking at age differences in strategic planning on the Tower of London (rather than in time to first move), we find
a similar pattern of age differences in task performance and, more importantly, that younger individuals perform worse than adults both because

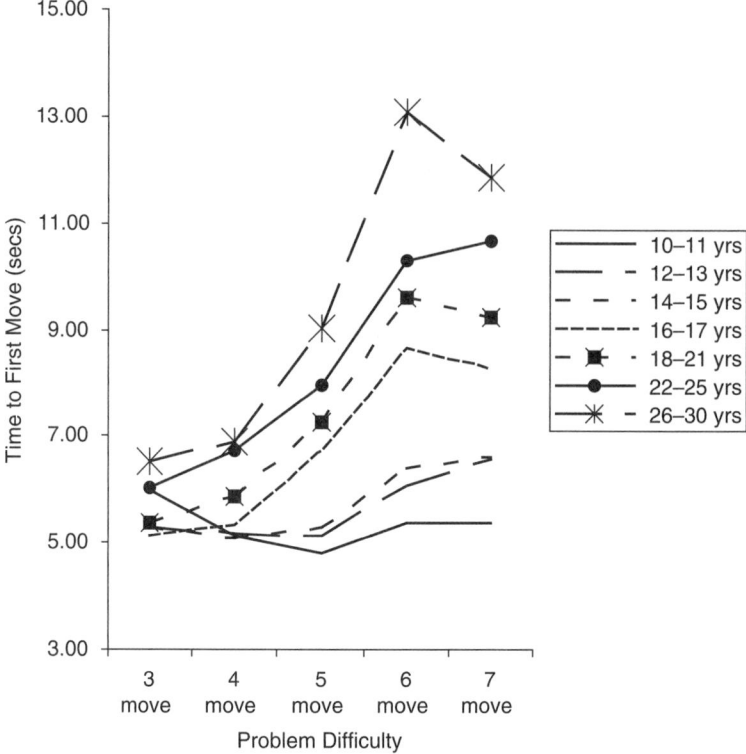

FIGURE 3.2. Age differences in time to first move on the Tower of London task as a function of problem difficulty.

Note: Means adjusted for IQ and SES. The age by problem difficulty interaction is significant at p < .001 (Steinberg et al., 2008).

of deficiencies in working memory and because of poorer impulse control (Albert & Steinberg, in press).

We used two tasks to examine age differences in reward seeking: the IGT and a delay discounting task. To examine age differences in reward seeking on the IGT, we examined change over time in draws from the advantageous and disadvantageous decks; recall that in our modified version of the task, these variables are independent, because participants can opt to not play at all when presented with a specific deck. Our hypothesis that reward seeking peaks in mid-adolescence was tested via two regression analyses (one predicting change in pulls from good decks between the first and last blocks of the task and one predicting change in pulls from bad decks); in each, as we did in our analysis of the self-reports of reward seeking, we entered

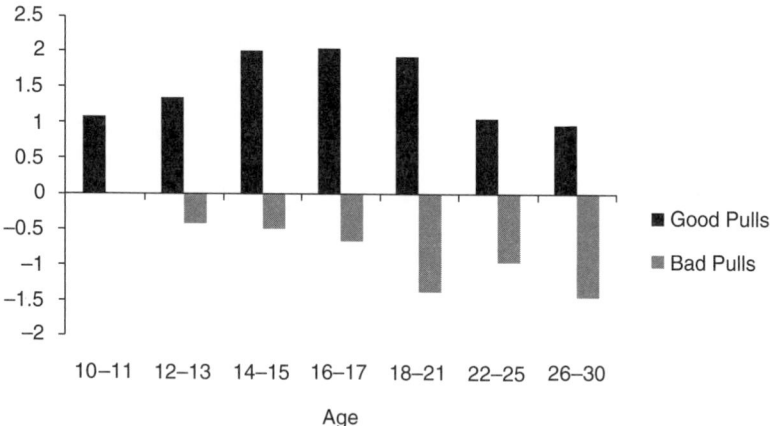

FIGURE 3.3. Age differences in changes over time in pulls from advantageous and disadvantageous decks in the Iowa Gambling Task.
Note: Means adjusted for IQ and SES. The curvilinear trend for advantageous pulls is significant at $p < .001$; the linear trend is not significant. The linear trend for disadvantageous pulls is significant at $p < .001$; the curvilinear trend is not significant (Cauffman et al., 2010).

age, IQ, and SES on the first step of the regression and the quadratic term for age on the second. As expected, and consistent with self-reports, draws from the advantageous decks increase between early and mid-adolescence and then decline between mid-adolescence and adulthood; the linear term is not significant ($\text{ß} = -.024$, ns) but the curvilinear term is significant ($\text{ß} = -.577$, $p < .001$). In contrast, in the prediction of change in pulls from the bad decks, only a pattern of linear change over time is shown, with individuals becoming more cost-averse with age ($\text{ß} = -.114$, $p < .001$); the quadratic term is not significant ($\text{ß} = .051$, ns) (see Figure 3.3). We also analyzed these data using multilevel modeling and came to the same conclusion (Cauffman et al., 2010).

The pattern of age differences shown in Figure 3.3 is striking. The bars indicate change in advantageous (black bars) and disadvantageous (gray bars) choices between the first and final blocks of the task; bars above the midline indicate an absolute increase in card pulls, whereas bars below the midline indicate a decrease. Among younger individuals, there is virtually no change over the course of the task in their pulls from bad decks, suggesting that they are paying little attention to costs; indeed, during the first half of adolescence, changes in card choices are almost entirely due to changes in the way that individuals respond to rewards. Among the adults,

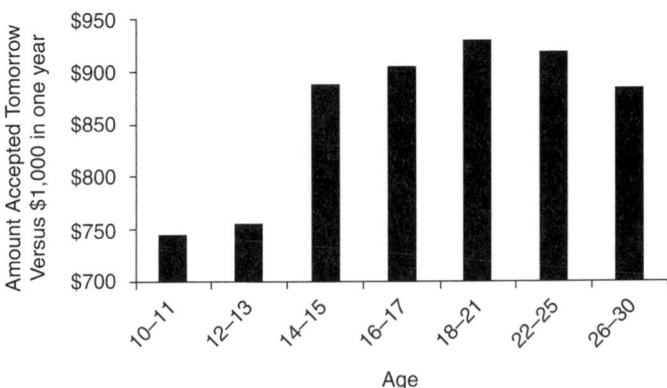

FIGURE 3.4. Age differences in delay discounting.
Note: Means adjusted for IQ and SES.

however, it appears that both rewards and costs are driving changes in performance over time.

Our findings on age differences in delay discounting suggest that it is not only rewards, but immediate rewards that influence the decision making of younger adolescents. As noted earlier, in the delay discounting paradigm, individuals are asked to choose between a delayed reward and an immediate one of lesser value. The so-called indifference point is the amount at which the subjective value of the short-term reward is equivalent to that of the delayed reward. Individuals who are willing to accept a smaller reward because it is delivered sooner have a lower indifference point.

An ANCOVA was conducted with age, gender, and ethnicity as between-subjects factors; IQ and SES as covariates; and individuals' indifference points at the six time intervals (one day, one week, one month, three months, six months, and one year) as the within-subjects factors. As in virtually all studies of delay discounting, we find a main effect of the repeated time factor (Greenhouse-Geisser $F(5,3555) = 6.64$, $p < .001$), indicating that individuals' indifference points decline as the delay interval increases. However, we also find significant age differences in average indifference points ($F(6,832) = 5.90$, $p < .001$), with younger individuals demonstrating lower indifference points – that is, stronger preference for immediate rewards – than older ones.

Figure 3.4 illustrates age differences in indifference point, using as an example the amount individuals would accept immediately rather than wait one year for $1,000. As the figure indicates, there is a dramatic break point around age fourteen or fifteen, with individuals thirteen and younger generally reporting lower indifference points than individuals sixteen and older, and individuals fourteen and fifteen falling somewhere in between. In fact, there are no significant age differences in average indifference points among individuals sixteen and older and no differences between the ten- and eleven-year-olds and the twelve- and thirteen-year-olds. Similar age differences are observed with respect to other delay intervals (Steinberg et al., 2009).

Taken together, the results of these analyses provide strong support for the dual-systems model of risk taking discussed earlier in the chapter. Reward sensitivity, preference for immediate rewards, and self-reported sensation seeking follow an inverted U-shaped function, increasing between preadolescence and mid-adolescence, peaking between the ages of fourteen and sixteen, and then declining. In contrast, self-reported impulse control as well as nonhasty behavior and strategic planning increase linearly from preadolescence through late adolescence.

CONCLUDING COMMENTS

According to their own reports, and as reflected in their performance on computer tasks designed to measure reward seeking and impulsivity, adolescents and adults differ in ways that are theoretically coherent with recent research on adolescent brain development, which points to extensive and dramatic remodeling of reward circuitry early in adolescence but a lengthier period of more gradual maturation of brain systems implicated in self-regulation (see Steinberg, 2010). Consistent with this neurobiological evidence, we find that heightened reward seeking, along with heightened attraction to immediate rewards, is most clearly and consistently seen during early and mid-adolescence. In contrast, gains in impulse control occur throughout adolescence and well into young adulthood.

The observed pattern of age differences on the self-report and performance measures of impulsivity were very similar, with both indicating a linear decline in impulsivity between ages ten and thirty. Similarly, the self-report and performance measures of reward seeking both showed the predicted relationship between reward seeking and age, with reward seeking increasing most during early adolescence.

The contribution of the present research to the literature on psychological development in adolescence and young adulthood stems from its inclusion of a much wider age range than has been examined previously in one sample (from age ten to thirty), its use of both self-report and cognitive-behavioral indicators of reward seeking and impulsivity, its socioeconomically and ethnically diverse sample, and its independent measurement of two constructs that often have been conflated both conceptually and empirically. The fact that differential patterns of age differences found in self-reports are similar to those found in conceptually linked behavioral tasks inspires more confidence in the conclusion that the developmental trajectories of reward seeking and impulsivity differ. Although one must be cautious about drawing inferences about change over time from cross-sectional research, the current findings provide a foundation from which further longitudinal study, using self-reports, behavioral tasks, and brain imaging, should proceed.

The heightened reward seeking and preference for immediate rewards during the first part of adolescence seen here calls to mind other studies of sensation seeking (e.g., Stephenson et al., 2003) and reward sensitivity (e.g., Galvan et al., 2006), which show increases in both during the early adolescent years; these increases are thought to be linked to increases and then declines in prefrontal and paralimbic dopamanergic activity during the period following puberty (Steinberg, 2008). To our knowledge, only one previous study (Galvan et al., 2007) has examined age differences in self-reported impulsivity over an age range comparable to that studied here. The linear decline in self-reported impulsivity seen across the entire age span we studied is consistent with the Galvan et al., (2007) investigation and with findings reported in studies of self-reported impulsivity that have included middle adolescents and adults (e.g., Leshem & Glicksohn, 2007). Our finding of a linear decline in hasty behavior on the Tower of London is consistent with previous studies using this paradigm (e.g., Asato et al., 2006); numerous behavioral studies that compare children, adolescents, and adults on a range of self-regulatory tasks such as the antisaccade, Flanker, Go/ No-Go, and Stroop (see Casey et al., 2008); and strong evidence of structural and functional maturation over the course of adolescence and well into the twenties of brain regions that subserve impulse control and other aspects of self-regulation (see Paus, 2009). Thus, converging evidence from self-report, behavioral, and neurobiological studies indicates that impulse control improves not only between childhood and adolescence, but also between adolescence and adulthood.

Aristotle (350 B.C./1954) famously observed that youth "are hot-tempered, and quick-tempered, and apt to give way to their anger," and there is a long history of anecdotal evidence, empirical investigation, and actuarial analysis indicating that adolescence is a time of heightened risk taking and recklessness (Steinberg, 2008). One impetus for the present study was to better understand developmental differences in factors believed to contribute to this pattern. Although opportunity factors (e.g., less vigilant parental monitoring, legal driving privileges, the availability of sex partners) undoubtedly influence the extent to which individuals actually take risks (Byrnes, 1998), most indicators of risk taking (reckless driving, delinquent behavior, attempted suicide, substance abuse, unprotected sex) follow an inverted U-shaped pattern over the course of individual development, with risky behavior generally higher in middle or late adolescence than in pre-adolescence or adulthood.

To the extent that vulnerability to risk taking is the product of high reward seeking and low impulse control, the findings of the present study suggest why risk taking may follow this inverted U-shaped pattern. The first half of the adolescent decade – between the ages of ten and fifteen – appears to be a time of growing vulnerability to risky behavior, as this period is characterized by relatively higher reward seeking and attraction to immediate rewards in the context of relatively lower impulse control; heightened reward seeking impels adolescents toward risky activity, and immature self-regulatory capabilities do not restrain this impulse. As to the other side of the inverted U function, vulnerability toward risky behavior would be expected to decline from age fifteen on, given that both reward seeking and impulsivity diminish after this age.

The research reported here suggests that vulnerability to the attractiveness of immediate rewards during early and middle adolescence is likely to be normative, which poses a challenge to those interested in the health and well-being of this age group. It is important to remember, however, that individuals of the same age vary in their reward seeking and impulse control, and that variations in these characteristics are related to variations in risky and antisocial behavior (Steinberg, 2008). Understanding how contextual factors influence the development of reward seeking and self-regulation, as well as the neural underpinnings of these processes, should be a high priority for those interested in the physical and psychological well being of young people.

REFERENCES

Albert, D., & Steinberg, L. (in press). Age differences in strategic planning as indexed by the Tower of London. *Child Development.*

(2011). Judgment and decision making in adolescence. *Journal of Research on Adolescence, 21,* 211–224.

Aristotle. (350 B.C./1954). *Rhetoric.* (W. Rhys Roberts, trans.). Available online at http://www.classics.mit.edu/Aristotle/rhetoric.html

Asato, M., Sweeney, J., & Luna, B. (2006). Cognitive processes in the development of TOL performance. *Neuropsychologia, 44*, 2259–2269.

Bearman, P., Jones, J., & Udry, J. R. (1997). *The national longitudinal study of adolescent health: Research design.* Chapel Hill, NC: Carolina Population Center.

Bechara, A., Damasio, A. R., Damasio, H., & Anderson, S. W. (1994). Insensitivity to future consequences following damage to human prefrontal cortex. *Cognition, 50*(1–3), 7–15.

Berg, W., & Byrd, D. (2002). The Tower of London spatial problem solving task: Enhancing clinical and research implementation. *Journal of Experimental and Clinical Neuropsychology, 25*, 586–604.

Beyth-Marom, R., Austin, L., Fischoff, B., Palmgren, C., & Jacobs-Quadrel, M. (1993). Perceived consequences of risky behaviors: Adults and adolescents. *Developmental Psychology, 29*, 549–563.

Byrnes, J. (1998). *The nature and development of risk-taking.* Hillsdale, NJ: Erlbaum.

Casey, B. J., Getz, S., & Galvan, A. (2008). The adolescent brain. *Developmental Review, 28*, 62–77.

Cauffman, E., Shulman, E., Steinberg, L., Claus, E., Banich, M., Graham, S., & Woolard, J. (2010). Age differences in affective decision making as indexed by performance on the Iowa Gambling Task. *Developmental Psychology, 46*, 193–207.

Centers for Disease Control and Prevention. (2006).Youth Risk Behavior Surveillance – United States, 2005. *Morbidity & Mortality Weekly Report, 55*(SS-5), 1–108.

Dahl, R. (2004). Adolescent brain development: A period of vulnerabilities and opportunities. *Annals of the New York Academy of Sciences, 1021*, 1–22.

Ennett, S., Tobler, N., Ringwalt, C., & Flewelling, R. (1994). How effective is drug abuse resistance education? A meta-analysis of Project DARE outcome evaluations. *American Journal of Public Health, 84*, 1394–1401.

Galvan, A., Hare, T., Parra, C., Penn, J., Voss, H., Glover, G., & Casey, B. J. (2006). Earlier development of the accumbens relative to orbitofrontal cortex might underlie risk-taking behavior in adolescents. *Journal of Neuroscience, 26*, 6885–6892.

Galvan, A., Hare, T., Voss, H., Glover, G., & Casey, B. J. (2007). Risk-taking and the adolescent brain: Who is at risk? *Developmental Science, 10*, F8–F14.

Green, L., Myerson, J., & Macaux, E. (2005). Temporal discounting when the choice is between two delayed rewards. *Journal of Experimental Psychology, 31*, 1121–1133.

Hein, K. (1988). *Issues in adolescent health: An overview.* Washington, DC: Carnegie Council on Adolescent Development.

Keating, D. (2004). Cognitive and brain development. In R. Lerner & L. Steinberg (Eds.), *Handbook of adolescent psychology* (2nd ed.). (pp. 45–84). New York: Wiley.

Leshem, R., & Glicksohn, J. (2007). The construct of impulsivity revisited. *Personality and Individual Differences, 43*, 681–691.

Martin, C. A., Logan, T. K., Leukefeld, C., Millich, R., Omar, H., & Clayton, R. (2001). Adolescent and young adult substance use: Association with sensation seeking, self-esteem and retrospective report of early pubertal onset. A preliminary examination. *International Journal of Adolescent Medicine and Health, 13*, 211–219.

Millstein, S., & Halpern-Felsher, B. (2002). Perceptions of risk and vulnerability. *Journal of Adolescent Health, 31S*, 10–27.

Morse, S. (2006). Brain overclaim and criminal responsibility: A diagnostic note. *Ohio State Journal of Criminal Law, 3*, 397–412.

National Research Council. (2007). *Preventing teen motor crashes: Contributions from the behavioral and social sciences.* Washington, DC: National Academy Press.

Ohmura, Y., Takahashi, T., Kitamura, N., & Wehr, P. (2006). Three-month stability of delay and probability discounting measures. *Experimental and Clinical Psychopharmacology, 14*, 318–328.

Ozer, E., & Irwin, C. (2009). Adolescent and young adult health: From basic health status to clinical interventions. In R. Lerner & L. Steinberg (Eds.), *Handbook of adolescent psychology* (3rd ed., Vol. 1, pp. 618–641). New York: Wiley.

Patton J., Stanford, M., & Barratt, E. (1995). Factor structure of the Barratt Impulsiveness Scale. *Journal of Clinical Psychology, 51*, 768–774.

Paus, T. (2009). Brain development. In R. Lerner & L. Steinberg (Eds.), *Handbook of adolescent psychology* (3rd ed., Vol. 1., pp. 95–115). New York: Wiley.

Peters, E., & Slovic, P. (2000). The springs of action: Affective and analytical information processing in choice. *Personality and Social Psychology Bulletin, 26*(12), 1465–1475.

Psychological Corporation (1999). *Wechsler abbreviated scale of intelligence.* San Antonio, TX: Psychological Corporation.

Reyna, V. F., & Farley, F. (2006). Risk and rationality in adolescent decision-making: Implications for theory, practice, and public policy. *Psychological Science in the Public Interest, 7*, 1–44.

Rivers, S., Reyna, V., & Mills, B. (2008). Risk taking under the influence: A fuzzy-trace theory of emotion in adolescence. *Developmental Review, 28*, 107–144.

Sisk, C., & Foster, D. (2004). The neural basis of puberty and adolescence. *Nature Neuroscience, 7*, 1040–1047.

Spear, P. (2000). The adolescent brain and age-related behavioral manifestations. *Neuroscience and Biobehavioral Reviews, 24*, 417–463.

Stanford, M. S., Greve, K. W., Boudreaux, J. K., Mathias, C. W., & Brumbelow, J. L. (1996). Impulsiveness and risk-taking behavior: Comparison of high-school and college students using the Barratt Impulsiveness Scale. *Personality and Individual Differences, 21*, 1073–1075.

Steinberg, L. (2004). Risk-taking in adolescence: What changes, and why? *Annals of the New York Academy of Sciences, 1021*, 51–58.

   (2007). Risk-taking in adolescence: New perspectives from brain and behavioral science. *Current Directions in Psychological Science, 16*, 55–59.

   (2008). A social neuroscience perspective on adolescent risk-taking. *Developmental Review, 28*, 78–106.

   (2009). Should the science of adolescent brain development inform public policy? *American Psychologist, 64*, 739–750.

   (2010). A behavioral scientist looks at the science of adolescent brain development. *Brain and Cognition, 72*, 160–164.

Steinberg, L., Albert, D., Cauffman, E., Banich, M., Graham, S., & Woolard, J. (2008). Age differences in sensation seeking and impulsivity as indexed by behavior and self-report: Evidence for a dual systems model. *Developmental Psychology, 44,* 1764–1778.

Steinberg, L., & Cauffman, E. (1996). Maturity of judgment in adolescence: Psychosocial factors in adolescent decision making. *Law and Human Behavior, 20,* 249–272.

Steinberg, L., Dahl, R., Keating, D., Kupfer, D., Masten, A., & Pine, D. (2006). Psychopathology in adolescence: Integrating affective neuroscience with the study of context. In D. Cicchetti & D. Cohen (Eds.), *Developmental psychopathology, Vol. 2: Developmental neuroscience* (pp. 710–741). New York: Wiley.

Steinberg, L., Graham, S., O'Brien, L., Woolard, J., Cauffman, E., & Banich, M. (2009). Age differences in future orientation and delay discounting. *Child Development, 80,* 28–44.

Stephenson, M. T., Hoyle, R. H., Palmgreen, P., & Slater, M. D. (2003). Brief measures of sensation seeking for screening and large-scale surveys. *Drug and Alcohol Dependence, 72,* 279–286.

Teicher, M., Andersen, S., & Hostetter, Jr., J. (1995). Evidence for dopamine receptor pruning between adolescence and adulthood in striatum but not nucleus accumbens. *Developmental Brain Research, 89,* 167–172.

Thompson-Schill, S. (2002). Neuroimaging studies of semantic memory: Inferring "how" from "where." *Neuropsychologia, 41,* 280–292.

Trenholm, C., Devaney, B., Fortson, K., Quay, L., Wheeler, J., & Clark, M. (2007). *Impacts of four Title V, Section 510 abstinence education programs.* Princeton, NJ: Mathematica Policy Research.

Weisberg, D., Keil, F., Goodstein, J., Rawson, E., & Gray, J. (2008). The seductive allure of neuroscience explanations. *Journal of Cognitive Neuroscience, 20*(3), 470–477.

Zuckerman, M., Buchsbaum, M. S., & Murphy, D. L. (1980). Sensation seeking and its biological correlates. *Psychological Bulletin, 88,* 187–214.

Zuckerman, M., Eysenck, S., & Eysenck, H. J. (1978). Sensation seeking in England and America: Cross-cultural, age, and sex comparisons. *Journal of Consulting and Clinical Psychology, 46,* 139–149.

4

What Are the Cognitive Skills Adolescents Need for Life in the Twenty-First Century?

DEANNA KUHN AND AMANDA HOLMAN

Teachers College, Columbia University

For many years, Inhelder and Piaget's (1958) theoretical framework has served as a guide for examining cognitive changes emerging during the second decade of life. More recently, excitement has been generated by the identification of developments in the brain through the second decade that may be implicated in cognitive changes that occur during this decade (see Keating, 2004; Kuhn, 2006, 2009, for review). Yet the concepts of adolescent thinking becoming more formal, more abstract, and/or more systematic have yet to be firmly anchored in the day-to-day realities of how adolescents think about matters of consequence to them and how they need to think in order to engage effectively in the modern world (Kuhn, 2008). Moreover, most of the empirical evidence related to adolescent cognitive skills does not present a picture of strong and secure competence, making the question of how to support cognitive development in adolescence a pressing one.

In the first part of this chapter, we identify three areas of cognitive competence that we argue are critical to adolescents' development if they are to engage optimally in twenty-first-century society. In the second part of the chapter, we describe some of our own efforts to support such development through the design of curricula to develop cognitive skills during what we argue is the critical period of early adolescence.

BECOMING MULTIPLE-CAUSE THINKERS

The lion's share of research on adolescent cognitive development has been devoted to acquisition of the control-of-variables strategy, which many but not all of those assessed exhibit mastery of by mid-adolescence. Indeed, skill in executing a controlled experiment, in which all variables except the one being manipulated are held constant so as to identify its effect on an outcome, has become a focus of process-oriented science curriculum beginning in the mid-elementary grades (NRC, 1996). Because the design of controlled experiments rarely stands out as an objective except in science classes, it has nonetheless remained unclear exactly how this capability affects thinking more broadly. Moreover, another aspect of coordinating multiple variables, one that we believe has profound consequences for everyday thinking, has until recently received little attention.

We refer to recognition of the fact that most outcomes in the real world are contributed to by multiple variables. To achieve a nuanced understanding of any such outcome, it is essential that this multiple causality be recognized and examined. Yet many people, the studies we have conducted show, are satisfied to identify a single causal factor as the explanation for an event and are disinclined to probe further. Why did their favored candidate win (or lose) the election? A single-cause explanation is likely to suffice in their thinking about the phenomenon, to the detriment of a richer understanding of the phenomenon and its place in the context of a myriad of interrelated events.

To investigate this phenomenon, we conducted a series of studies in which we asked children, adolescents, and adults to predict outcomes for specific cases for which they had identified a status on multiple antecedent variables that had been shown to contribute to the outcome (Kuhn & Dean, 2004; Kuhn, 2007; Kuhn, Iordanou, Pease, & Wirkala, 2008; Kuhn, Pease, & Wirkala, 2009). Although they were in agreement that each of these antecedent variables affected the outcome, the task proved surprisingly difficult at all age levels. When, after making an outcome prediction for a specific case, we asked which of the antecedent variables had figured in their prediction (see example in Figure 4.1), they often mentioned only one or two, fewer than the number they had earlier identified as relevant. Although performance improved with age and education, even many adults performed poorly in this respect. The assumption is clearly unwarranted, then, that once students are able to perform controlled experiments, they will have no difficulty in applying this skill to identify and coordinate the simultaneous effects of multiple variables on an outcome.

In studies with sixth-graders, we therefore explored potential sources of difficulty with this task. The first source we were able to discount was keeping in mind the various contributing factors that had been identified as affecting an outcome. Even when we provided pictorial memory aides depicting the various effects, these response patterns persisted (Kuhn et al., 2008). Performance does improve with practice over time (Kuhn et al., 2009), but the weaknesses are persistent and do not disappear entirely. In

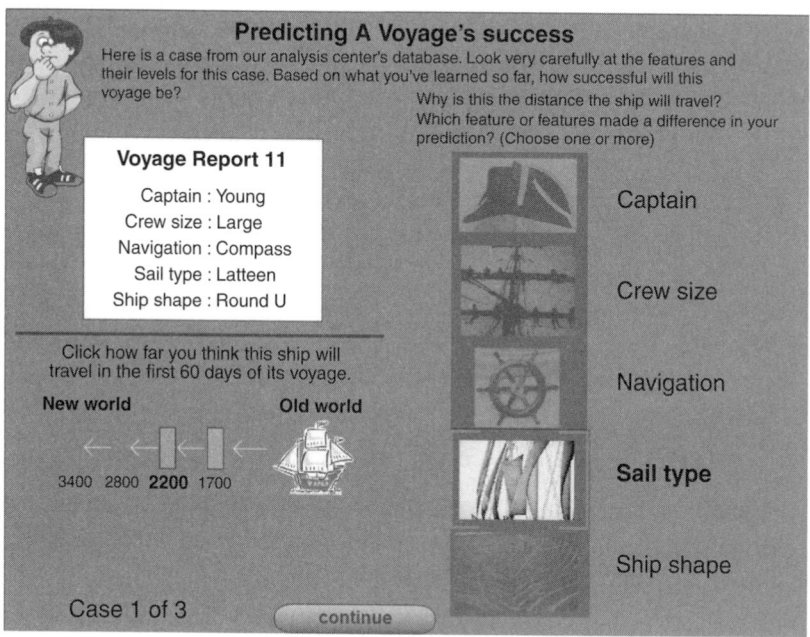

FIGURE 4.1. Sample prediction task.

particular, we observed a common conceptual error that is crucial in scientific reasoning, a confusion between the levels of a variable and the variable itself. Thus, a frequent response to the question of which variables had affected a prediction judgment was, for example, "I considered the snake activity, because it's high and that increases [earthquake] risk, but I didn't consider any of the others because they were all low so they wouldn't matter." What the student in this case does not recognize is that, unlike the noncausal variables, the other two causal variables of course had to be considered, or she would not have been able to categorize their levels as ones associated with lower risk. They could not be ignored.

Students of this age appear to have at best a fragile concept of what a variable is, without which it is difficult to reason explicitly or with precision about the effect of one variable on another. In particular, the concept that under consistent conditions a variable operates in a consistent way across occasions is fundamental to science, and yet it is a concept that children appear to only gradually acquire, and one therefore that cannot be assumed to be in place. Equally fundamental to science is the assumption that to be adequately explained, most events require a confluence of multiple causes to be invoked. In the absence of this assumption, scientific thinking is severely constrained. Variables and multiple causation are the bread and butter of science. Despite their often being taken for granted in the design of science curricula, our studies suggest that neither of these assumptions is easy to come by.

Beyond the science classroom, the implications of adolescents' remaining "one-cause" thinkers into and through adulthood have not been widely discussed but are profound. One-cause thinkers are confined to thinking simplistically. They cannot, or at least habitually do not, mentally represent the complexity of the ways in which events in the real world are interrelated. Early adolescence, we believe, is a critical period in which to seek to develop the competencies and dispositions that support multiple-cause thinking.

ENTERING THE WORLD OF INTELLECTUAL DISCOURSE

Another set of competencies and dispositions that we see as equally critical to begin supporting in early adolescence are similarly ones that have until recently received relatively little attention in the study of adolescent cognition. We refer to argumentive discourse and reasoning, which traditionally have been overlooked by researchers in favor of the study of individual problem solving – long the focus of attention in research on reasoning in cognitive psychology. Yet argumentation can be regarded as the umbrella under which all reasoning falls (Oaksford, Chater, & Hahn, 2008) – asserting, supporting, and refuting claims is the purpose to which we apply our reasoning skills.

Do adolescents need support if they are to become proficient arguers? The numerous assessments of high school students' writing are consistent in showing their skills to be weak at best in expository essay writing. Such assessments leave it unclear the degree to which challenges in writing versus thinking explain their poor performance. Thinking in real-world contexts is most importantly a social skill. It is in contributions to purposeful interactions with others that thinking skills are likely to have their greatest impact. For this and some other reasons, we have focused our study of developing argument skills on argumentive discourse. Dialogic argumentation has long been of broad interest to developmentalists who regard social collaboration as central to cognitive development (Damon, 1984; Smetana, Killen, & Turiel, 1991; Moshman, 2005). Argumentative discourse, we and others (Billig, 1987; Kuhn, 1991; Graff, 2003) have proposed offers a promising path to the development of the individual skills in verbal and written expository argument that become increasingly critical with age in academic settings. Among its strongest virtues from a developmental perspective are its roots in young children's everyday conversations. A familiar activity – everyday talk – has the developmental potential to with exercise develop into an unfamiliar one – formal expository writing. In Graff's (2003) terms, dialogic argument provides the "missing interlocutor" that makes individual argument difficult and, for many students, seem even pointless. Adolescents constantly engage in spirited discourse with peers. Can we channel that competence in fruitful directions?

In our studies of young adolescents' dialogic argumentation on contemporary social issues (Kuhn, Shaw, & Felton, 1997; Felton & Kuhn, 2001; Kuhn & Udell, 2003; Felton, 2004; Udell, 2007), we have found that most focus their efforts on exposition of their own position to the neglect of attending to the opponents' claims and attempting to weaken their force – what, along with securing commitments to support one's own claims, Walton (1989) identifies as the two basic goals of skilled argumentive discourse. Yet when explicitly instructed to do so, they are able to attend to the opponent's argument and even generate counterarguments against it (Kuhn & Udell, 2007). When explicitly asked to give a reason against the opposing position, the large majority of sixth- and seventh-graders that we describe in this chapter were able to do so. When asked simply, however, "What is the best argument to make?" only a minority mention the opposing position and identify weaknesses in it. Thus, at least as important as developing the skill of constructing counterarguments to weaken the opponent's claims is recognizing the need to do so.

Our intervention studies, in which we engage young adolescents in extended practice in engaging in argumentive discourse with their peers (Kuhn & Udell, 2003; Felton, 2004; Udell, 2007; Kuhn, Goh, Iordanou, & Shaenfield, 2008), have shown that argumentation skills do advance with practice in ways that we are able to measure. Before turning to a description of our argument curriculum, however, we note our findings with respect to a third, and closely related, achievement of critical importance to adolescent cognitive development.

VALUING DISCOURSE

Because our studies of argument skills early on told us that teens may display more competence, when explicitly asked to do so, than they habitually exercise, we have given as much attention to disposition as to competence in our research. Doing so has brought us directly to the study of intellectual values, as well as their underpinnings in epistemological understanding. Kuhn and Park (2005) presented questions like these to adolescents:

> Many social issues, like the death penalty, gun control, or medical care, are pretty much matters of personal opinion, and there is no basis for saying that one person's opinion is any better than another's. So there's not much point in people having discussions about these kinds of issues. Do you agree, somewhat agree, or disagree?

Although variability was high across cultures, many teens agreed, giving such reasons as "It's not worth it to discuss because it's not something you can get a definite answer to," or "There's no point because you're not going to get anywhere; everyone has a right to think what they want to." These responses point to the foundation that intellectual values have in epistemological understandings of what it means to know. Adolescence is the characteristic time at which we see a shift from an understanding of knowledge as certain and accumulating to the radical relativism – the ubiquitous "whatever" stance that is the typical product of adolescents' efforts to cope with the discovery of the uncertainty of knowledge (even on the part of so-called experts; Moshman, 2005, 2008; Kuhn, 2009).

If adolescents are to regard intellectual discourse as worth the effort it entails, they must see the point of it. Otherwise, they are not going to be disposed to involve themselves in it in any deep way. Doing so requires progressing beyond the relativist's stance that any opinion is as good as any other to the recognition that some opinions have more merit than others, to the extent they are judgments supported in a framework of argument and evidence.

Kuhn, Wang, and Li (in press) probed teens regarding two specific scenarios, both ones in which we would hope them to recognize the value of discourse – one that offers the opportunity to enhance understanding through discourse and the other in which discourse is essential to achieve a goal. The scenarios were as follows:

Collaborative opportunity scenario. Two candidates, Bo and Le, are running for governor of your state. You are riding the bus with your friend. You know your friend prefers Bo. You prefer Le. Is it a good idea to discuss Bo and Le with your friend?

Collaborative necessity scenario. The director asks your three-person team to develop a new product that will do a better job than the old one and to send a report when you've finished. Your teammate B has an idea of what to do, but you have an idea that you think is better. Teammate C has no ideas. What should you do to start? Describe your plan.

(Follow-up question) It turns out that you and B have a big disagreement. B thinks his idea is best and you think yours is best. What should you do?

The most frequent response of eighty American sixth-graders to the opportunity scenario was that the topic should not be discussed – 41 percent gave this response. The remainder said the topic should be discussed and divided almost equally into the two subcategories with respect to their justifications. Only 30 percent of the sample both endorsed discussion and gave justifications indicating that the purpose of such discussion would be to enhance understanding. The remaining 29 percent of the sample endorsed discussion but saw its purpose as communication (of one another's positions) and, for some, the potential to cause one person to change their position. Illustrations of responses in each of these categories appear in Table 4.1. Because the reasons for not engaging in discussion are of particular interest, each of the range of different reasons that appeared in this category is illustrated, although the large majority (69% of this category) fell into the category of concern about risk of argument (33%) and jeopardizing of friendship (36%). No differences appeared across gender.

Response categories and illustrations for the necessity scenario appear in Table 4.2. These appear in approximate increasing order of sophistication, an ordering devised only for the purpose of coding in cases in which a respondent offered multiple solutions at different points in their response to the scenario. In these cases, the response was classified as falling into the most advanced of the category types the respondent invoked. Again, no gender differences appeared.

Comparison across the two tables shows that endorsement of discussion as an opportunity (first scenario) and as a strategy for achieving a goal (second scenario) occur with nearly the same frequency across the two scenarios – among slightly less than one-third of respondents.

The responses of young teens in this study and the study by Kuhn and Park (2005) told us that if we were going to work at developing the argument skills of adolescents, we would have to work at least as hard on disposition as on competence. That recognition is reflected in the argument curriculum that we now describe.

AN ARGUMENT CURRICULUM FOR MIDDLE SCHOOLERS

The argument curriculum we describe here has evolved over several iterations, but the goals and broad strategies have remained constant. We target

TABLE 4.1. *Sixth-graders' responses to the opportunity scenario*

Category	Examples
Don't Discuss (41%)	
It's not interesting	"I don't like talking about government with my friends. Usually we talk about movies and rockstars."
It serves no purpose	"No, because it's my opinion so I wouldn't discuss it to change my friend's opinion because it's his own thought."
	"They can think whatever they want. I don't want to change their opinion about it. We can be friends and have different interests."
It risks argument	"You could get into an argument."
	"Because it's a personal opinion and it can lead to disagreements."
It risks argument and jeopardizes friendship	"Because it could ruin your friendship."
	"You could get into a serious argument and you may not be friends anymore. Also, if you don't, arguments can be avoided and your friendship has a better chance of being longer."
	"Your friend might feel disrespected and might not want to be your friend anymore."
Discuss to Communicate or Influence (29%)	"You'll see why the other likes the person they prefer and you can show them the same."
	"You can convince him to like Le so you can like the same candidate."
Discuss to Understand (30%)	"Because she might know more about the other candidate and I might know more about the one I'm for. We could tell each other more and we would learn something new. Although we might get into a fight, if we were both nice we wouldn't."
	"Because if you discuss the candidates' pros and cons, you might see that either you or your friend is for the wrong person and might want to change sides."
	"If we talk about it we might be able to come to a conclusion."

specific argumentation strategies that we believe are key ones in which adolescents must develop skill. At the same time, however, we seek to develop the intellectual values that will enable teens to see these strategies as having a productive purpose – as worth the effort they entail. Third, by engaging teens in deep and focused discussion of difficult social issues, we endeavor to enhance their understanding of the complexity of such issues – that they

TABLE 4.2. *Sixth-graders' responses to the necessity scenario*

Category	Percent of responses	Examples
Prevail by power	08%	"I would try to persuade him to say my idea is the best."
		"Bring other people to help you out that would support your opinion."
Defer to another	28%	"Let C decide."
		"Go with B's idea so he doesn't get mad."
		"Tell the director if you can't work it out."
Search for an alternative	05%	"Find an idea we both like and use that one."
		"Brainstorm and come up with something better."
Combine	26%	"Combine both of your ideas."
Compare via test	05%	"Test his idea first, then test mine."
		"Try to do both ideas and see who does it better."
Discuss	28%	"We should debate and see problems to both of our ideas."
		"Have a group discussion where we all share our thoughts and ideas. We would vote and discuss how some ideas are better. Then we will all agree on one."

cannot be conceived of in terms of the one-factor causes or solutions that we noted earlier as typical at this age level.

Our approach rests on the claim underlying all of our microgenetic research (Kuhn, 1995) – that dense exercise of existing strategies over a period of time is quite often a sufficient condition for change. Two features of this exercise that we believe are critical in all contexts are, first, that this exercise be goal-directed – that is, that it have a purpose from the subject's point of view – and second, that it be designed so as to promote meta-level reflection on the activity rather than simply its performance. Our initial studies emphasized the first feature and our later ones the second. In current work, we have devised a way to incorporate both.

Assessment of each students' skill in dialogic argumentation occurs at the beginning and end of a year-long intervention. At each assessment, the student engages in one live debate with a classmate and one electronic debate with another classmate, each of whom holds an opposing view on a social issue. (At present, our assessment topics are capital punishment and euthanasia.) Reassessment is based on the same pair arguing the same topic at the later time. Skill assessment focuses on the extent to which the student directly addresses each of the opponent's claims, attempting to weaken it with a relevant counterargument. We also include measures of individual argumentative essay writing on a separate topic, as well as a recognition measure, involving a choice of which of two counterarguments to an argument is the stronger one.

The curriculum itself focuses on four topics that students engage over the course of the year, each over a sustained period of twice-weekly class sessions for seven to eight weeks. Students begin with topics close to their own experience and gradually move to social topics of broader scope. Engagement with each topic comprises three phases, which we refer to as the Pregame, the Game, and the Endgame. The first four sessions are devoted to the Pregame and emphasize the goal-directed aspect of the activity. Students meet in small groups of seven or eight, in which all share the same position on the topic and together form the team for that topic. Their task is to explore, evaluate, and organize arguments to support their position, as well as to anticipate their opponents' responses.

During the main Game phase, same-side students each work with a partner to engage in an electronically conducted dialog with a pair of students from the opposing side. The social collaboration with a partner in constructing responses to the opposition supports metacognitive reflection on the dialogic interchange. Also supporting this reflection are the transcripts of the electronic dialogs that remain visible for students to refer to, in contrast to spoken dialog, which disappears as soon as it is uttered. As a further support, while they are waiting for the opposing pair to respond, the pair of students collaborate on reflection sheets (Figure 4.2) that give them an opportunity to review and reflect on what has transpired. The idea that evidence is relevant to argument and essential in supporting and refuting claims and building strong arguments is gradually introduced with successive topics and plays an increasingly important role thereafter, as students increasingly take charge of identifying and seeking evidence that will strengthen their arguments and counterarguments.

Following the series of five to seven dialogs with a series of opposing pairs, students move to the Endgame phase by returning to their same-side small groups and beginning two sessions of preparation for a final "Showdown" – live full-group debate between the opposing sides. At the showdown, an A and a B teams on each side are formed, with A teams presiding during the first half of the showdown and the B teams playing a supportive role of making suggestions. During the second half, A and B teams switch roles. During the showdown, students on the presiding team organize themselves, with students taking turns in "Hotseat" interchange with a representative of the opposing side, punctuated by team-called "Huddles"

Team Members: _____ Date: _____

Let's think... starting with <u>OUR OWN</u> main argument:

> One of our main arguments was:
> _____
> _____
> _____

> Their counterargument to our main argument was:
> _____
> _____

> Our comeback was:
> _____
> _____

> How could our comeback be improved? Write a better, more effective comeback here:
> _____
> _____
> _____
> _____

Get the ball back over the net

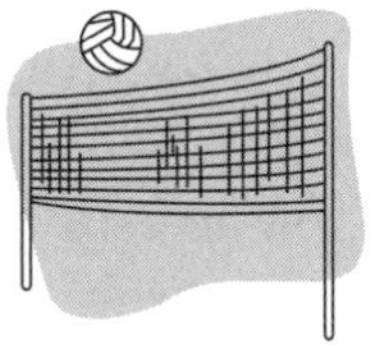

FIGURE 4.2. Sample reflection sheet.

to debate strategy. The sequence ends with reflective activities that include viewing a video of the showdown, evaluation of an Argument Map prepared for them based on the showdown debate, with scoring of strong and weak moves, and a final individual position essay that students write on the topic.

WHAT DEVELOPS?

We have now implemented an argumentation curriculum of the sort described among a range of young adolescent groups. The population from

which our examples here are drawn is an urban public middle-school population of mixed academic ability, ranging from below-average to acceler-
ated, and highly diverse ethnically and socioeconomically, but the method
has also proven successful with less able, severely academically disadvantaged populations, including residents in a juvenile detention facility
(DeFuccio, Kuhn, Udell, & Callender, 2009). In each case, we have evaluated the outcomes on a number of different dimensions.

STRATEGIC DEVELOPMENT: ADDRESSING
THE OTHER'S ARGUMENT

The first and most crucial development we look for is an increase in students' ability and willingness to attend critically to the other's argument.
Until this happens, no genuine argumentation has occurred. We have
observed two phases in this evolution. The first and most fundamental is
recognizing the need to attend to the other's argument and investing the
cognitive effort in doing so. The second is constructing a counterargument
that weakens the force of the other's argument. Not all counterarguments
have this characteristic. Students' early counterargument efforts very often
consist of disagreement with the opponent's statement but then followed
not by a critique of it but rather by an alternative argument against the
opponent's position that leaves the opponent's statement unaddressed. For
example, in his first dialog on the initial topic (Should a misbehaving student be expelled from school?), one boy was confronted with his opponent's statement, "They shouldn't be expelled because they deserve another
chance." His reply ignored his peer's "another chance" concept and instead
introduced a new, perfectly sound argument against the opponent's *position*, but one that leaves the opponent's *argument* intact: "Yes but they have
been acting up for a while and their behavior has not gotten better and it's
not fair to the other kids who are trying to learn."

Near the end of the year, in a dialog on the fourth topic (Should sale of
human organs be allowed?), the same boy exhibited greater skill in genuine counterargument. His opponent argued, "[They] shouldn't be allowed
to because it is part of their body," and this time he directly addressed and
undertook to weaken his opponent's argument: "But if people are willing to
give up their own body parts and be so generous to the people who need
kidneys why should we stop them …?"

These gains are reflected at a group level in Figures 4.3 and 4.4, which are
based on the progress of ninety-four sixth-graders across the school year in
which they participated in the program. Figure 4.3 shows the proportions

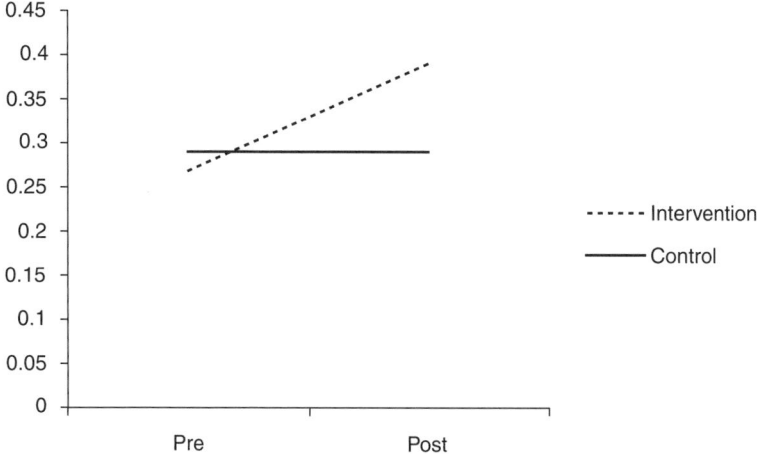

FIGURE 4.3. Proportion of utterances coded as direct counterarguments.

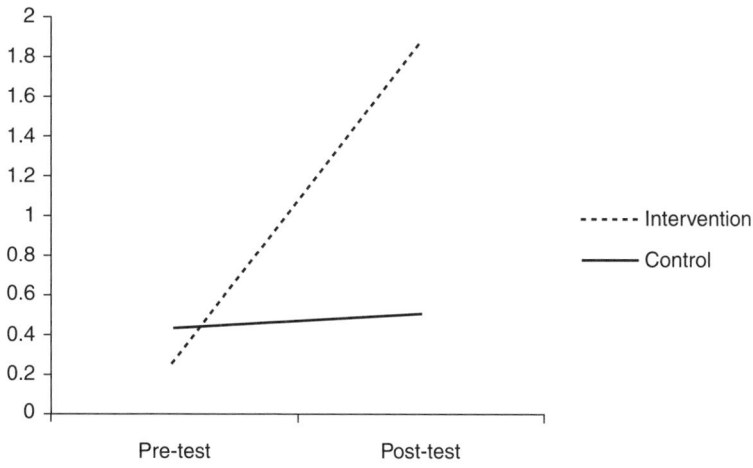

FIGURE 4.4. Rebuttal sequence lengths.

of their discourse utterances that were coded as direct counterarguments to the opponent's immediately preceding claim. Figure 4.4 reflects their skill in sustaining sequences of counterarguments – in other words, rebuttal. As shown, these sequences become longer over time.

The transition represented in Figures 4.3 and 4.4 reflects a transition from focus on one's own position and supporting arguments to a focus on the other's position and supporting arguments and how these should be addressed.

Once this important transition is underway, students are ready to address another fundamental component of skilled argumentation – evidence.

INTEGRATING EVIDENCE INTO ARGUMENT

In our argumentation curriculum for middle-school students, we initially do not identify for students the entity of evidence as one for them to be concerned about. Our rationale is to let students draw on their own knowledge base as they see fit and to focus their efforts on developing the practice of authentic discourse with a peer in which the other's contributions are attended to and addressed. After they have done so during the first year of the curriculum, at the end of the first and beginning of the second year, we introduce some evidence related to the topic they are discussing. We do so casually, mentioning that we have gathered some information that we are making available to them and that may be of use to them in their argumentation. This information takes the form of a set of questions (about eight to ten), each printed on the outside of an envelope, inside of which is printed on a card a two-to-three-sentence factual answer to the question. The set of envelopes is centrally located in the classroom, and students must go through a simple procedure of checking out and returning any envelope they wish to access.

The questions and answers are carefully chosen to reflect a range of relations to the two opposing positions being debated. A few fairly directly support one position and a few the other, but others do not clearly do either and might be invoked in connection with more than one primary or secondary claim. For the organ sale topic, for example, two of the questions were "How humanely are animals treated in laboratories?" and "Has animal testing led to cures for any human diseases?"

Initially, students show only slight interest in these evidence envelopes, but over time they access them more frequently, and we begin to see the appearance of the information they contain in students' discourse. At the same time, an even more interesting phenomenon gathers steam: One or two students ask if they can submit their own questions that they would like to have answered. This request is accepted, other students get interested in this possibility and begin to participate, and student-submitted questions and answers become part of the evidence base available for student use. Over subsequent topics, student-generated questions become so plentiful that the need for researcher-generated questions becomes minimal, and these are reduced to one or two introduced at the beginning to get the process started. A final phase of this process occurs when students take over

TABLE 4.3. *Questions posed by students during argumentation on the president topic*

How much does the U.S. spend on the Iraq war?

How many Americans have lost their jobs?

How many people have gone homeless because of America's [economic] crisis?

In the past how have economic crises been solved?

How have other presidents dealt with these issues?

How many economic crises have we had before?

How many Americans have died in the Iraq war?

What is the UN? What is their main job?

What is the U.S. or Obama doing about the economy; for example, how are they making money literally?

If any, what other countries are trying to help the U.S. out of its economic crisis?

Approximately how long will it take to bring home the military to America?

Why and how did the economy problem start?

What other serious international issues are there?

What else can we be spending the money on that we are spending on the war?

How much debt are we in with all the countries?

How much money does the U.S. have? Do we have more than 3 trillion dollars?

How much money does the U.S. spend each day/week?

How long was the Great Depression?

How did we get out of the Great Depression?

What kinds of extreme things can happen when people lose their job?

What [private] foundations are there that help with the economy?

Which issue is taking up the most money in our budget?

What is water pollution doing to the people and animals that live in/eat/drink it?

How much did George Bush focus on global warming?

How much money will it take Obama to fix the economic crisis?

Compared to other countries, how bad is the economic condition in the U.S.?

How do problems in the U.S. directly affect other countries?

Did the U.S. ever make a promise to always help other countries?

How many alliances does the U.S. have with other countries; what are those countries?

Will helping other countries help us gather alliances?

How can alliances help us fix the problems of the nation?

for themselves not only question generation but generation of answers to their own questions. This is a phase with which we are just beginning to experiment, although it is clearly the desired endpoint in terms of an idealized practice.

In Table 4.3 appear many of the wide array of questions that one group of seventh-grade students generated as they addressed the topic of whether the newly elected president should focus his effort on domestic or international issues. These questions and answers came to figure strongly in their argumentation. We see this evolution toward evidence seeking and incorporation into argument as significant on multiple grounds. At a strategic level, clearly argumentation is enriched. But at least as important is the epistemological advancement that this evolution represents. These were all questions that students themselves identified as ones they wanted the answers to, because they believed that answers to them would facilitate their argumentation. Their recognition of their importance signifies two kinds of epistemological advance – one with respect to strategy and the other concerning content. With respect to strategy, these students have begun to appreciate the role of evidence in argument. With respect to content, they have begun to appreciate the complexity of and subtleties of the issues they are discussing, a development we address in more detail shortly.

We are now studying how students make use of evidence in their argumentation and how their strategies in coordinating claims and evidence evolve with practice. The two core strategies we observe are the Support strategy (using the evidence to support one's own claim) and the Challenge strategy (using the evidence to challenge the other's claim). Also, however, we begin to see additional types of talk *about* the evidence and its functions. These are particularly important because they entail meta-level statements about evidence (and, implicitly at least, its status in relation to a claim). The simplest is a defensive statement supporting the validity of the evidence that has been used as support for one's own claim: "We know this from one of our evidence cards." Although the relation is most often not explicitly stated, such statements occur in conjunction with a claim and it is implicit that the evidence, if accepted, will serve to bolster the claim. What we see much less frequently is a parallel invocation of evidence with the goal of weakening the other's claim – a strategy we have reason to think may be a more challenging and cognitively advanced achievement. What we do see, however, are attempts to discredit evidence the other has introduced "That doesn't prove anything," or, quite often, to criticize the lack of evidence. The phrase "You don't have any proof" becomes a common refrain. Or, "You would know this if you looked at the evidence." Or, more charitably, evidence may be solicited: "Do you have evidence to prove that?" These are all, of course, from an epistemological perspective extremely important contributions to the discourse, in as much as they reflect a recognition and endorsement of shared norms of discourse.

TRANSFER ACROSS DOMAINS AND TO INDIVIDUAL
EXPOSITORY ARGUMENT

At the beginning and end of a year-long intervention, students engage in dialogs on a topic that has not been part of the curriculum. Hence we are able to show that their progress occurs in argumentation skill more broadly and is not confined to the particular topics about which they have argued. Transfer was also evident when the curriculum topic was scientific in nature and the assessment topic social-scientific, and vice versa (Iordanou, in press). Similarly, Udell (2007) found that teen girls showed transfer from a topic of personal importance (teen pregnancy) to a less personally relevant social issue (capital punishment), and vice versa. Thus, there is evidence that developing the relevant skills in a particular domain, be it social, scientific, or personal, allows transfer of skills to other domains.

Another highly desirable outcome of our argument curriculum would be to witness students applying these argumentation skills in their individual writing. Students show a considerable lack of skill in individual written argument when assessed by standardized tests (NAEP, 2007), despite the fact that the ability to write a persuasive essay is roundly considered an important educational outcome. As noted earlier, Graff (2003) posits that argumentive writing gains purpose and clarity when the writer accesses an internal argumentive discourse with an imagined interlocutor who the writer then attempts to convince in his or her writing. We believe that practicing argumentation with a peer, as students do in our program, promotes this process in two ways. First, the practice students get in anticipating, attending to, and countering the opponent's arguments implicitly strengthens an internal interlocutor as the agent to whom the written argument is directed. Second, by coming to recognize the importance of directly countering one's opponent in discourse, the writer will eventually achieve this same recognition in the written mode.

Although our analyses of these developments in individual written work are still underway, there is indication that such transfer is indeed occurring. Students' individual written essays on the pretest and posttest (non-intervention) topic were superior on multiple dimensions among students who participated in the year-long curriculum, compared to a group who did not (Kuhn et al., 2008). Our current work suggests this is true as well for a fresh essay topic that is not the subject of any dialogic interchange.

TABLE 4.4. *Reflections on the value of argument*

What have you learned this year?

How to argue without getting mad or frustrated.

I've learned how to argue without screaming and fighting with someone. I've learned
that by screaming and shouting you don't get your point across because you are
making the person concentrate on your anger; but by speaking they
can understand you and analyze your idea.

I've learned to listen to what other people are saying and then really counter it.

I've learned to make strong arguments and be sure to use evidence.

Somebody is a lot more willing to listen and to agree with what you have to say if you
back it up with reasons.

We should think a little more before we respond so that we can have better
constructed responses.

We should learn to clarify our statements so our opponents don't get confused.

I've learned you need to have backup and good reasoning to win ... to weaken their
argument.

One skill I've learned is counter, which is when you counter back to what the person
said, not getting off topic. Another is to listen to what the person is saying &
arguing straight to the argument, weakening the counter that was said to you.

I've learned that when you assume something will happen but you are not exactly
sure if it will or not, it is called an unwarranted assumption.

To counter reasons that people have and to give a good reason back. This is a good
method in your daily life to use when you are in a crisis.

Having a skill to argue for something effectively is important because it helps you be
able to write better essays (which are basically just arguments in writing).

EPISTEMOLOGICAL ACHIEVEMENTS

What do students who participate in our curriculum learn *about* argumentation? A sample of their responses, when we asked them directly what
they had learned in the class, is presented in Table 4.4. As these responses
reflect, students' awareness of gains covers a broad spectrum. They include
learning to contain emotion, to listen, to think, to provide reasons to support claims, and to respond directly to what the other has said. All of these
reflect shared intellectual values that are every bit as important as the skills
needed to practice them. Explicit awareness of skills ("I've learned to listen
to what other people are saying and then really counter it") is particularly
important as it is a necessary first step toward meta-level management and
regulation of their use. The responses in Table 4.4 also suggest an encouraging developing awareness of where and when these skills will be useful.

A further very encouraging indication of epistemological achievement
has to do with the content of students' claims. In eliciting their positions

on topics, we also asked how certain they were that their position was the correct one. Students in both intervention and comparison groups tended to express high certainty in initial assessments. Among the intervention group, however, this certainty – on the very same topic – declined. In the comparison (non-intervention) group, by contrast, it increased slightly.

CONCLUSION

The decreasing certainty just noted, and the epistemological advance that it reflects, offers a point of convergence across the three strands of development we have traced here – coming to appreciate the authentic complexity of most phenomena, making them unsuited to single-cause explanation, coming to recognize the purpose and value of intellectual discourse, and developing the intellectual skills that provide entry into the realm of ideas, analysis, and discourse. Most of the most important things people know they do not know with certainty. Yet they are still worth knowing, by which we mean worth holding up to continuing scrutiny and evaluation. And most knowing is fundamentally social in nature, meaning it requires scrutiny in the dialogic context of discourse with others who bring multiple points of view to the discussion. But repeatedly, we find, a great many adults are inappropriately certain about what they know, and, as the data presented here suggest, even among those in higher education settings, many have not come to appreciate the role that intellectual discourse plays in advancing human knowing.

If we wish to prepare our young people for their roles as citizens in the twenty-first century – roles in which we cannot predict precisely what they individually and collectively will need to know – we need to do all we can to support their coming to engage in and value the practices needed to participate in communities of intellectual discourse. Many have written about all that is wrong with the way we educate adolescents. An essential step in righting it is to identify what it is that they need to know and know how to do, in terms they can find convincing. We would like to think that the work described here is a contribution in that direction.

REFERENCES

Billig, M. (1987). *Arguing and thinking: A rhetorical approach to social psychology.* Cambridge: Cambridge University Press.

Damon, W. (1984). Peer education: The untapped potential. *Journal of Applied Developmental Psychology* 5(4), 331–343.

DeFuccio, M., Kuhn, D., Udell, W., & Callender, K. (2009). Developing argument skills in severely disadvantaged adolescent males in a residential setting. *Applied Developmental Science, 13*, 30–41.

Felton, M. (2004). The development of discourse strategies in adolescent argumentation. *Cognitive Development, 19*, 35–52.

Felton, M., & Kuhn, D. (2001). The development of argumentive discourse skills. *Discourse Processes, 32*, 135–153.

Graff, G. (2003). *Clueless in academe: How schooling obscures the life of the mind.* New Haven, CT: Yale University Press.

Inhelder, B., & Piaget, J. (1958). *The growth of logical thinking from childhood to adolescence.* New York: Basic Books.

Iordanou, K. (In press). Developing argument skills across scientific and social domains. *Journal of Cognition and Development.*

Keating, D. (2004). Cognitive and brain development. In R.M. Lerner, & L. Steinberg (Eds.), *Handbook of adolescent psychology* (2nd ed., pp. 45–84). Hoboken, NJ: John Wiley & Sons.

Kuhn, D. (1991). *The skills of argument.* New York: Cambridge University Press.

(1995). Microgenetic study of change: What has it told us? *Psychological Science, 6*, 133–139.

(2006). Do cognitive changes accompany developments in the adolescent brain? *Perspectives on Psychological Science, 1*, 59–67.

(2008). Formal operations from a twenty-first century perspective. *Human Development, 51*, 48–55.

(2009). Adolescent thinking. In R. Lerner & L. Steinberg (Eds.), *Handbook of adolescent psychology* (3rd ed.). Hoboken NJ: Wiley.

Kuhn, D., & Dean, D. (2004). Connecting scientific reasoning and causal inference. *Journal of Cognition and Development, 5*, 261–288.

Kuhn, D., Goh, W., Iordanou, K., & Shaenfield, D. (2008). Arguing on the computer: A microgenetic study of developing argument skills in a computer-supported environment. *Child Development, 79*(5), 1310–1328.

Kuhn, D., Iordanou, K., Pease, M., & Wirkala, C. (2008). Beyond control of variables: What needs to develop to achieve skilled scientific thinking? *Cognitive Development, 23*, 435–451. [Special issue, The Development of Scientific Thinking, B. Sodian & M. Bullock, eds.]

Kuhn, D., & Park S. (2005). Epistemological understanding and the development of intellectual values. *International Journal of Educational Research, 43*(3), 111–124.

Kuhn, D., Pease, M., & Wirkala, C. (in press). Coordinating effects of multiple variables: A skill fundamental to causal and scientific reasoning. *Journal of Experimental Child Psychology.*

Kuhn, D., Shaw, V., & Felton, M. (1997). Effects of dyadic interaction on argumentive reasoning. *Cognition and Instruction, 15*(3), 287–315.

Kuhn, D., & Udell, W. (2003). The development of argument skills. *Child Development, 74*(5), 1245–1260.

(2007). Coordinating own and other perspectives in argument. *Thinking and Reasoning, 13*, 90–104.

Kuhn, D., Wang, Y., & Li, H. (in press). Why argue? Developing understanding of the purposes and values of argumentive discourse. *Discourse Processes*.

Moshman, D. (2005). *Adolescent psychological development: Rationality, morality; and identity* (2nd ed.). Mahwah NJ: Erlbaum.

——— (2008). Epistemic development and the perils of Pluto. In M. Shaughnessy, M. Vennman, & C. K. Kennedy (Eds.), *Metacognition: A recent review of research, theory and perspectives* (pp. 161–174). Hauppauge, NY: Nova.

NAEP. (2007). The Nations Report Card: Writing 2007, National State and Trial Urban Districts. Retrieved December 13, 2008 from NAEP Web site: http://nces.ed.gov/nationsreportcard/pdf/main2007/2008468.pdf

National Research Council (1996). *National science education standards.* Washington, DC: National Academies Press.

Oaksford, M., Chater, N., & Hahn, U. (2008). Human reasoning and argumentation: The probabilistic approach. In J. Adler & L. Rips (Eds.), *Reasoning: Studies of human inference and its foundations*. New York: Cambridge University Press.

Smetana, J., Killen, M., & Turiel, E. (1991). Children's reasoning about interpersonal and moral conflicts. *Child Development, 62*, 629–644.

Udell, W. (2007). Enhancing adolescent girls' argument skills in reasoning about personal and non-personal decisions. *Cognitive Development, 22*(3), 341–352.

Walton, D. N. (1989). Dialogue theory for critical thinking. *Argumentation, 3*, 169–184.

5

Hypothetical Thinking in Adolescence: Its Nature, Development, and Applications

ERIC AMSEL

Weber State University

It is the mark of an intelligent mind to be able to
entertain an idea without necessarily accepting it.
– Aristotle

Classic theories of human development characterize adolescence as a period of an awakening of new, powerful, and pervasive abilities and talents. Such was the claim of G. Stanley Hall (1904, cited in Grinder 1969, p. 358) who noted that "adolescence is … the only point of departure for the superanthropoid that man is to become." Similarly, Piaget (1972; Inhelder & Piaget, 1958) held that adolescence is the period in which new and powerful forms of reasoning emerge. These abilities and talents are so novel that both G. Stanley Hall (1904; and, see Grinder, 1969) and Jean Piaget (Piaget, 1972; Inhelder & Piaget, 1958) identify a context and a period of time for the nascent adult to cultivate these skills. These abilities are so encompassing that they are thought to result in fundamental changes in how teens think, forever transforming their views of themselves, others, and the world (Erikson, 1968; Kohlberg, 1984; Selman, 1980).

In this chapter, I explore hypothetical thinking as one of the novel, powerful, and pervasive achievements of adolescence that fundamentally impacts and alters them. Specifically, I examine the nature of hypothetical thinking, its process of development, and applications in the life of adolescents. Hypothetical thinking places a premium on what Aristotle cited as the mark of an intelligent mind – the ability to entertain an idea without necessarily accepting it. Central to hypothetical thinking is the ability to assume, suppose, or stipulate as true claims that may conflict with what is accepted as true about the world. The ability to treat ideas *as if* they were true is implicated in a variety of significant human endeavors, from systematically testing a hypothesis, logically reasoning about an argument, constructing a possible world, regretting one's life choices, or reacting to a pretend enactment. These examples point to one of the most curious things about hypothetical reasoning. It is implicated in spontaneous and playful pursuits such as pretense, and in formal and serious intellectual activities such as logic or science.

THE NATURE OF HYPOTHETICAL THINKING

Hypothetical thinking is defined as the ability to reason about alternatives to the way the world is believed to be (Rescher, 1961, 1964; St. B. T. Evans, 2007). The definition highlights three general components: recruiting the imagination, making inferences about imagined states of affairs, and interpreting the real-world consequences of the states imagined. Hypothetical thinking as the process of generating hypotheses, arguments, fictions, alternative event sequences, or pretend scenarios involves the *imagination*. The imagination is used to create alternatives to reality that are distinguished from reality. These alternative states of affairs may be represented in mental models and are created by imagining variations or mutations of accepted beliefs about reality, thereby contravening those beliefs.

Hypothetical reasoning also requires making *inferences* about the imagined states of affairs. For example, outcomes can be inferred from the constructed mental model of an alternative world, with its belief-contravening claims. The inferential process may range from formally drawing conclusions from premises whose truth status is either known to be false, unknown, or indeterminate (Rescher, 1961, 1964), or by literally running the mental model of an alternative world through a process known as *mental simulation*. Mental simulations exploit real-world causal knowledge to actually put into motion the conditions specified in the mental model of an alternative world and then to read off its outcome (Kahneman & Tversky, 1982). However it is accomplished, the inferential process in hypothetical reasoning provides a basis to understand possible outcomes of alternative worlds.

Finally, considering alternatives to the way the world is believed to be involves *interpretations* of the differences between the worlds believed to be true and the imagined alternative one. At very least, this means keeping track of differences between the claims made about the two different worlds, but it may also mean that the outcome of the alternative world is used to understand the meaning and significance of events that do occur. For example, discovering how an alternative action may have led to a better outcome than the one resulting from a person's actual actions may result in the person experiencing regret (Landsman, 1993). Alternatively, discovering how the alternative actions of a person would have made no difference in a negative outcome may relieve the person of responsibility for the outcome. In both cases, actual events are evaluated in light of imagined alternative ones that might have occurred.

FORMAL OPERATIONS AND HYPOTHETICAL REASONING

The central thesis of the chapter, that hypothetical reasoning is a transformative ability acquired in adolescence, is not new. Piaget made this point more than fifty years ago and revisited this topic over the years (1972; 1987; Inhelder & Piaget, 1958). According to Piaget (1972), adolescents acquire the ability to form hypotheses about reality and test them out. Such an ability, he claimed (Piaget, 1972, p. 3), is "the principle novelty of the period" and is "a decisive turning point because to reason hypothetically and to deduce consequences that the hypotheses necessarily imply (independent of the truth or falsity of the premise) is a formal reasoning process." Inhelder and Piaget (1958) understood hypothetical reasoning as reflecting the operation of an underlying formal hypothetico-deductive system that allows the adolescent to anticipate *all* logical possibilities in a situation. Inhelder and Piaget (1958) documented both the underlying formal system and the actual reasoning of children and adolescents on tasks requiring them to identify factors influencing various physical phenomena (e.g., buoyancy, pendulum periods, material flexibility, acceleration, chemical reactions). Only adolescents approached the tasks by systematically generating and testing out hypotheses rather than just subjectively acting on the apparatus or exploring empirical relations operating in the apparatus. Piaget (1972) later recognized that hypothetical reasoning does not emerge fully formed and universally applicable in adolescence, but is demonstrated first in domains of personal interest and relevance. Even later, Piaget (1987) further acknowledged that the ability to entertain possibilities is not just the product of the growth of reasoning from childhood to adolescence, but also the motor of that development as children expand their horizons about the widening set of possibilities out of which reality springs (also see Gallagher & Reid, 1981).

To Piaget what is unique about adolescence is that the imagination becomes under the control of an abstract logical system, giving hypothetical reasoning the status of an objective and systematic tool by which to consider possibilities. Young children's reasoning about possibilities is subjective and unsystematic, derived from and limited to their real-world knowledge, beliefs, and activities. However, adolescents become able to reason objectively and systematically about possibilities, resulting in them inverting the relationship between the real and possible such that there is a "subordination of the real to the realm of the possible" (Piaget, 1972, p. 3; also see Mueller, Sokol, & Overton, 1999).

Consider combinatorial reasoning, the ability to generate all possible combinations of *n* elements. When *n* is small, even young children can work though all combinations using their domain knowledge, experience, or trial and error (English, 1993). But as the value of *n* increases, it becomes more difficult to compute all combinations without an ability to think logically about possibilities (Dimant & Bearison, 1991). Combinatorial reasoning is among the first formal operations skills acquired (Broughton, 1983; Robarge & Flexer, 1979), reflecting adolescents' grasp of the logic underlying possibilities and laying the foundation for the acquisition of other logico-mathematical reasoning skills (Moshman, 1998; Robarge & Flexer, 1980).

A number of criticisms have been leveled at Piaget's claim that adolescents become capable of logical (i.e., objective and systematic) reasoning about possibilities. The first is that even adults struggle to reason hypothetically in this manner. It is difficult for many adults to reason about possibilities without being inappropriately influenced by what they know, believe, or desire about a situation. From this perspective, hypothetical thinking is hard work, requiring the careful and conscious regulation of available beliefs, knowledge, and desires in order to reason about possibilities in an unbiased manner (Kuhn, 2001; St. B. T. Evans, 2007). On the other hand, hypothetical thinking can be as easy as child's play. Young children's pretend play has been characterized as creating and reasoning about alternative worlds (Carruthers, 2002; Nichols & Stich, 2000), which taps the same ability to reason about possibilities as any other form of hypothetical or creative thinking (Carruthers, 2002). Both these criticisms assert that hypothetical thinking, in the form of objective and systematic reasoning about possibilities, is neither acquired nor perfected by adolescents, undermining the central thesis of the chapter. I review each of these criticisms with an eye to understanding what it is about hypothetical reasoning that is uniquely acquired during adolescence.

HYPOTHETICAL THINKING AS CHILD'S PLAY

While pretending that an empty cup is full of tea, a two-year-old child turns over the cup, spilling its imaginary contents onto a teddy bear. When asked, the toddler describes the cup as now being empty and proceeds to clean up the imaginary mess with a rag. Such a scenario was documented by Harris and Kavanaugh (1993) as part of their exploration of the extent to which two-year-olds' pretend play involves creating and reasoning about imagined alternatives to the way the world is. Harris and Kavanaugh, like others, were convinced of the capacity for the youngest of children to reason according to the three characteristics of hypothetical thinking previously described: recruiting the imagination, making inferences about imagined states of affairs, and interpreting the real-world consequences of the states imagined. First, young children use their imagination to create alternatives to the way the world is believed to be. In the scenario documented above, young children treated an empty cup *as if* it were filled with water. Second, inferences were readily made regarding the consequences of the imagined features of the cup. The pretending child correctly inferred not only that a mess would result if a cup full of water were overturned, but also correctly inferred precisely where the mess would be. Finally, the child kept track of the differences between the claims made about a pretend and real world[1] and made sure that there were *no* consequences for beliefs about the real world of entertaining an imagined pretend world. This latter point is important, as profound conceptual confusion results if the pretend world influences children's interpretation of real-world beliefs (Leslie, 1987). For example, conceptual chaos results if pretending that a banana is a telephone alters a child's real world concept of bananas to include the features and functions of telephones.

Young children's ability to both generate alternatives to reality and appreciate their implications and consequences has led many to characterize pretense as a form of hypothetical reasoning in which children act consistently with respect to pretend claims (Amsel, 2000; Amsel, Bobadilla, Coch, & Remy, 1996; Harris, 2000; Harris & Kavanaugh, 1993; Leslie, 1987; Lillard, 2001; Nichols & Stich, 2000; Perner, 1991). This is a completely different characterization of pretense than Piaget's (1962). For Piaget (1962), pretense is a form of egocentric and maladaptive thinking in which reality is largely assimilated to the idiosyncratic and subjective desires and wishes of the child, with no corresponding alteration of mental structures to accommodate reality (see Harris, 2000). The claim that pretense is intrinsically a form of hypothetical reasoning challenges Piaget's account of the very trajectory of cognitive development itself. To Piaget, development proceeds from the subjective and idiosyncratic forms of thinking represented by pretend play to the objective and unbiased forms of thinking represented by formal reasoning about possibilities. The Piagetian account of development collapses

---

[1] Claims about the pretend world are designated as *pretend claims* and claims about the real world are designated as *belief claims*.

onto itself if in pretend play young children can demonstrate their ability to use hypothetical thinking as an objective and systematic tool for understanding possibilities.

Although there is agreement that pretend play implicates a form of hypothetical reasoning, there is less agreement on the kind of achievement it signifies. Leslie (Friedman & Leslie, 2007; Leslie, 1987) proposes that belief claims are encoded in a first-order representational system that takes input from the world, such as the claim that *a cup is empty*. Pretend claims are encoded in a metarepresentational system that takes propositions from the first ordered system after they are copied, edited, and attached to an agent who is identified as pretending. So a child pretending the empty cup is full of water represents that *I* (agent) *pretend* (operator) *that the "empty cup contains water"* (copied and edited first-order proposition).

Others propose that pretense involves an agent treating pretend claims *as if* they were true, requiring no metarepresentation of an agent or the pretend claims. One proposal is that children represent the belief and pretend claims together in a counterfactual proposition that is flagged or marked as pretend (Harris & Kavanaugh, 1993; Nichols & Stich, 2000). For example, Nichols and Stich (2000) propose that a pretending child represents the proposition *this [empty] cup contains water*, in a *possible world box*, which is a special cognitive workspace that marks the proposition and related ones as counterfactual. Another proposal is that children represent relevant belief and pretend claims in distinct models and then coordinate the two (Lillard, 2001; Perner, 1991; Perner, Baker, & Hutton, 1994). For example, Perner (1991) assumes two distinct cognitive models of a pretend situation, one encoding beliefs claims (e.g., REAL: *this cup is empty*) and the other encoding pretend claims (HYPOTHETICAL: *this cup contains water*).

In research addressing the cognitive representations underlying pretense, Amsel et al. (1996) had three-year-olds identify the actions (combing), and the actual (a fork) and pretend (a comb) identities of objects used in an episode of pretense (pretending to comb hair with a fork). These identifications were made as children observed another's pretense or recalled their own initial pretense activities in multiple pretense scenarios. Although they had little difficulty identifying the actions performed, the children were more likely to correctly identify the actual than the pretend identity of the object (also see Albertson & Shore, 2008 and Wyman, Rakoczy, & Tomasello, 2009). Interestingly, there was no contingency in correctly identifying the objects' identities, as would be expected if children form a single representation encoding together both belief and pretend claims. The findings were interpreted as suggesting that underlying young children's pretense is their representation of the pretend and the real worlds in distinct models (Amsel et al., 1996; Amsel & Smalley, 2000).

There is no reason to think that only two models of the world exist at any given time. Weisberg and Bloom (2009) found that children may form multiple distinct models for different pretend worlds. They found that pre-schoolers who created a particular pretend identity for an object in one pretend scenario would not spontaneously use the same object for the same pretend function in a second pretend scenario that was occurring simulta-neous to or after the first scenario. It seems that children form boundaries between multiple pretend worlds, a finding replicated in their understand-ing of fictional worlds (Skolnick & Bloom, 2006).

It appears that pretense involves some but not all cognitive skills that are central to hypothetical thinking. The hypothetical thinking skills impli-cated in pretense include creating a model of an alternative to world that is distinguished from real world. The boundary between the worlds is porous enough for children to *import* real-world knowledge when necessary into the pretend world. But the boundary is largely impermeable to the child moving in the other direction so that real-world beliefs and knowledge remain unaffected by engaging in pretense.

However, pretense does not seem to require two critical components of hypothetical thinking. First, the form of hypothetical reasoning implicated in children's pretend play need not be objective and systematic in the sense of children creating a realistic or serious *possible* world. Instead, children's pretend worlds may be fanciful, reflecting a process of hypothetical think-ing that is subjective and idiosyncratic. Although a child may pretend that make-believe water pours from a glass in the pretend world in much the same way as it does in the real world, there is no guarantee that the child will pretend that the water will have all and only those properties it is believed to have in the real world. Children may not feel compelled to ensure that all features and processes of the real world are present in the pretend world. Second, the form of hypothetical thinking in pretend play does not require that children's understanding of the real world is affected by or subordi-nated to the pretend one. The evidence suggests that children readily keep the pretend and real worlds separate (Woolley, 1995, 1997). Although there are cases of "leakage" of the pretend world into the real world (Bourchier & Davis, 2002), such cases are best described as local and temporary failures rather than general and long-term vulnerabilities.

Although not tapped by pretend play, children may nonetheless have fledging abilities to objectively and systematically create alternative possi-ble worlds to reality, which are used to understand reality. In one line of research, children as young as two years of age have been shown to make valid deductions on counterfactual syllogism tasks simply by framing the counterfactual premise as make-believe (Amsel, Trionfi, & Campbell, 2005; Dias & Harris, 1988, 1990; Markovits & Vachon, 1989; Richards & Sanderson, 1999). For example, Amsel et al. (2005) found that when invited to *pretend* a make-believe world in which dogs meow, and introduced to Rover the dog while still pretending, six-year-olds tended to validly infer that Rover meows. Forty percent of the six-year-olds gave logically valid answers on all three make-believe trials, which is significantly above chance responding. The findings suggest that children are able to use logic to objectively and systematically guide inferences regarding the pretend world.

To test children's limitations to reason logically in a Make-believe condition, Amsel et al. (2005) included a Hypothetical condition that invited children to reason logically about counterfactual premises in an analog of a possible world. In the Hypothetical condition, participants were invited to *imagine* what the real would be like if dogs meow, then, while they were still imagining, were introduced to Rover the dog, and asked whether Rover meows. Only 17 percent of the six-year-olds gave logical answers on all three of the hypothetical trials, a percentage no different than expected by chance and significantly lower than the percentage consistently making valid judgments in the Make-believe condition. A ten-year-old group also demonstrated a disparity between the Hypothetical and Make-believe conditions, but this was erased among college students (see Figure 5.1). The results suggest that the children in the two younger groups have difficulty using logic to reason objectively and systematically about a counterfactual premise in a serious *possible* world compared to a fanciful *pretend* world.

Participants in Amsel et al. (2005) were also asked about the features of the alternative creatures they created in the Make-believe and Hypothetical conditions. Participants were asked whether the alternative creatures they imagined had features of the object and subject of the counterfactual claim. In the case of meowing dogs, participants were asked about whether the creature has two features of dogs (e.g., growls and wags its tail) and two features of cats (e.g., purrs and eats mice). Generally, participants' syllogism performance was consistent with their attribute judgments. Only participants who consistently made logically valid inferences in the Make-believe and Hypothetical conditions were selective about the features of their creatures. They affirmed more features of the objects (dog) than subjects (cat) of the counterfactual claim, seemingly reflecting on and evaluating the features that a hybrid animal might actually possess.

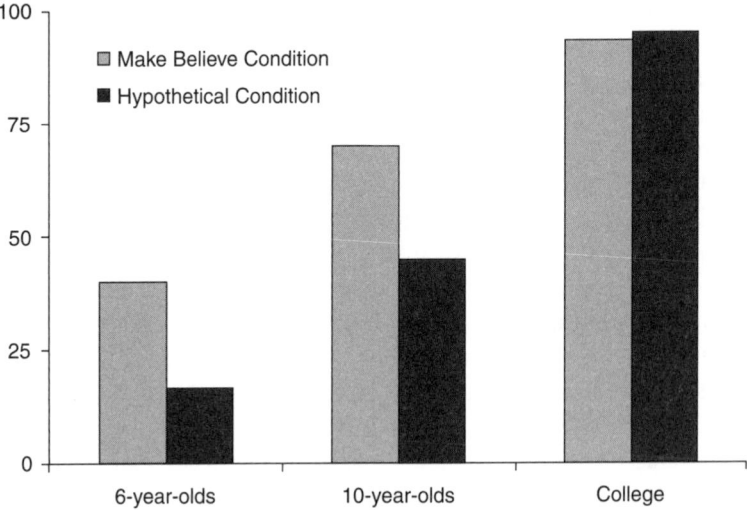

FIGURE 5.1. Percentage of consistently correct participants by instruction condition and age group in Amsel, Trionfi, and Campbell (2005), Study 2.

The importance of critical reflection on judging possibilities has recently been confirmed in a series of studies by Shtulman (2009; Shtulman & Carey, 2007). Despite an ability to distinguish real from pretend and ordinary from impossible states of affairs, children have difficulty distinguishing between improbable and impossible ones, denying that each is possible. Shtulman explains that children's modal judgments are based on whether they had first hand experiences of the events. In contrast, adults make modal judgments of impossibility by critically reflecting on and evaluating their experience of events against their causal knowledge to decide whether the event is in fact impossible or just improbable.

The role of critical reflection and evaluation of possible worlds is a central concern in another line of research on children's abilities to objectively and systematically think hypothetically. Generally, even young children have been shown to correctly answer future hypothetical questions of the sort, *what would happen if . . .* (Riggs, Peterson, Robinson, & Mitchell, 1998; Robinson & Beck, 2000). Children create and run a mental simulation in order to understand the future of a given state of affairs. However, they may not understand that for a given state of affairs, there may have been an alternative possibility that could have occurred instead. This latter ability has been tested in counterfactual reasoning research in which children are assessed for their ability to infer alternative possible event sequences, given hypothetical changes to the antecedent or consequence of the actual sequence (Amsel & Smalley, 2000; Guajardo, Parker, & Turley-Ames, 2009; Harris, German, & Mills, 1996; Riggs & Peterson, 2000; Riggs et al., 1998; Robinson & Beck, 2000). For example, Amsel & Smalley (2000) report a card game in which preschoolers and adults were given two face-down cards and had to choose one to turn over. If participants turned over a card with the highest number, they won the hand and earned stickers or small gifts. On trials where the participant turned over a losing card, they were invited to turn over the alternative card. On these trials, preschoolers, like adults, could readily understand that, although they lost the hand, they would have won the hand if only they had turned over the alternative card. This finding suggests that children can objectively and systematically create possible worlds that have consequences for understanding the causal role of events in the actual event sequences.

Beck, Robinson, Carroll, & Apperly (2006) and Rafetseder, Cristi-Vargas, and Perner (2010) questioned whether all appropriate controls were exercised on these counterfactual reasoning tasks. Beck et al. (2006) argued that perhaps children's responses on counterfactual reasoning tasks may not actually reflect an understanding of possible states of affair. In Beck et al. (2006, Study 2), preschoolers were presented with a slide in which a toy could take one of two routes. After seeing a toy take one route down the slide, they were asked two different questions. Although they could readily answer a question about alternative *outcomes*, typically requested in standard counterfactual tasks (*What if the toy had gone the other way, where would it be?*), they had more difficulty answering an open counterfactual question regarding alternative *possibilities* (*Could the toy have gone anywhere else?*). Beck and colleagues concluded that young children do not treat alternative outcomes as possibilities, which appears to require critically reflecting on different outcomes to appreciate their status as alternative possibilities.

Rafetseder et al. (2010) similarly found that previous research has over-estimated young children's counterfactual reasoning competence. They designed a task that minimized children's ability to use knowledge about general conditional relationships to answer the specific counterfactual questions without ever constructing a possible world. For example, perhaps children in Amsel et al.'s (2000) card game could answer counterfactual questions by using their general conditional knowledge about the game (if a high card is turned over, you win the game) without actually constructing an alternative possible world in which they turned over the other card. Rafetseder et al. (2010) found that adolescents and adults were able to reason counterfactually in conditions minimizing the use of general conditionals to answer counterfactual questions, although six-year-olds showed only a fledgling ability to do so.

The later onset view of counterfactual reasoning was also reported in the studies of the counterfactual emotion of regret. Regret is a negative counterfactual emotion based on appreciating that better outcomes would have been realized if only one had acted differently (Landman, 1993; Gilovich & Medvec, 1995). For example, consider a scenario that Guttentag and Ferrell (2004) presented to six-year-olds, seven-year-olds, and adults:

> Bob and David both ride their bikes to school each morning. There are two paths that go to school around a pond. You can ride along the red path or you can ride along the yellow path. Everyday, when Bob gets to the pond he goes along the red path around the pond. Today, Bob took his usual way to school along the red path. Unfortunately, today a tree fell across the red path. Bob hit the branch with his bike, fell off his bike, was hurt and was late for school. Everything on the yellow path was fine. David always goes along the yellow path. However, today David decided that instead of going along his usual yellow path to school he was going to ride along the red path. David also hit the tree, fell off his bike, was hurt and was late for school. Who would be more upset about deciding to ride along the red path around the pond that day?

Adults and seven-year-olds judged that David feels greater regret despite both protagonists being in exactly the same state of having been hurt by biking on the red route. David was judged as feeling more regret presumably because the accident is understood in light of a normally taken alternative route that would have avoided the accident. That is, reality is understood in light of possibilities that could (and perhaps should) have occurred, but did not. However, the group of six-year-olds did not judge that David felt worse than Bob. The pattern of results was explained by the failure of young children to relate actual states of affairs to counterfactual ones. Even if children create alternative possible worlds, they are not used to interpret actual event sequences.

This explanation was explicitly tested by Amsel and Smalley (2000), who used the card game task described previously. As noted, young preschoolers and adults readily recognized conditions in which they would have won the card game by engaging in alternative actions (i.e., turning over the other card). However, only adults were affected by discovering the value of the unchosen card. Adults but not preschoolers showed a change in their feelings recorded on a simple scale (ranging from very happy to very sad) before and after they discovered the alternative action would have resulted in a different outcome. This failure by children to relate factual and counterfactual states of affairs has been replicated by others (Beck & Crilly, 2009; McCloy & Strange, 2009), suggesting that young children lack a critical component of hypothetical thinking: the ability to interpret reality in light of possible alternatives to reality.

Young children's pretend play appears to include some important components of hypothetical thinking. They can readily create an alternative world and think logically with respect to it. Indeed, they may be able to create multiple imaginary worlds and keep each conceptually and ontological distinct (Skolnick & Bloom, 2006; Weisberg & Bloom, 2009). But these alternative imaginary worlds are not possible worlds by which reality can be understood. The general point – that young children do not appreciate imagined alternative worlds as *possible* ones – is echoed in the logical and counterfactual reasoning literatures. Moreover, research on regret reasoning suggests that the alternative worlds created by older children do not affect their evaluation of actual events. Children's challenge in creating and reasoning about serious *possible* worlds may lie in their ability to critically reflect on and evaluate the content of their alternative worlds. This was suggested from children's difficulty in reasoning logically about hypothetical premises, which was related to the unconstrained representations of the alternative worlds they created and modal reasoning literature, which points to children's lack of reflection to distinguish possible from impossible events.

HYPOTHETICAL THINKING AS HARD WORK

Although it is clear that young children have some of the component skills to reason hypothetically, the present section addresses whether adolescence is a time that component skills of hypothetical thinking are fully coordinated to function as an effective tool by which to understand reality in light of possibilities. If this view is correct, then adolescents should demonstrate the ability to objectively and systematically entertain, reason about, and interpret reality in light of possibilities across a variety of contexts and situations. Yet it is precisely this ability that appears to be a challenge to not only adolescents, but also adults. Even examining performance on complex combinatorial tasks as an index of objective and systematic reasoning about possibilities, adolescents and adults are challenged depending on the content and demands of the task (Fischbein & Gazit, 1988; White, 1985).

In this section, I review literatures that identify challenges that hypothetical reasoning poses to adolescents and adults. The first literature addresses the development and regulation of counterfactual emotions of regret. This work identifies regulatory challenges posed by directing the hypothetical thinking underlying regret, including limiting the influence of actual beliefs, knowledge, and desires. The second literature addresses the development and regulation of hypothesis testing that involves treating variables as possible causes or causal hypotheses of an outcome. Adolescents and adults are limited in entertaining theoretical beliefs as potentially false and in consciously coordinating theoretical beliefs and evidence. In both cases, adolescents' and adults' regulatory difficulties undermine their ability to effectively use hypothetical reasoning as an objective and systematic tool to understand reality in light of possibilities.

Returning to hypothetical reasoning and the experience of regret, consider being told a story about a protagonist choosing between one of two boxes and winning a *good* gift. But, in the box not chosen, there was a *great* gift, which the protagonist could have had if only she had chosen the alternative box. The story continues with the protagonist peeking into the box not chosen and discovering the better gift. It is easy to judge that the protagonist felt regretful that she had not chosen the other box, reflecting an understanding that receiving the good gift is only one possible way reality could have turned out. Such stories were presented to preschoolers, children, young adolescents, and adults (Guttentag & Ferrell, 2008). Everyone but the preschoolers judged that the protagonist felt regret, replicating previous work described earlier of the difficulty young children have with experiencing regret or understanding when it occurs. However, in another set of questions, Guttentag and Ferrell (2008) found that only a majority of adults were able to appreciate that a protagonist would want to avoid discovering the content of an unchosen box, thereby anticipating and seeking to avoid regret. Moreover, only the adolescent and adult groups expressed hope that the unchosen box was empty, again anticipating and seeking to avoid regret. The findings suggest that although children understand the conditions and contexts that result in regret, only adolescents begin to anticipate these conditions and contexts and think through ways to avoid regret. The hypothetical thinking necessary to *experience* regret is made that much more challenging when the regret is *anticipated*.

Even college students' ability to anticipate regret can be seen as fledging when the conditions put participants' desires into conflict with their ability to objectively and systematically reason hypothetically. Amsel, Cottrell, Sullivan, & Bowden (2005) assessed young adolescents (eleven-year-olds) and college students' ability to make decisions that avoid anticipated regret. Participants read about a protagonist making an everyday decision that put into conflict what the protagonist (and participants) would want to do with what they ought to do (i.e., studying for an exam or going to a movie with friends; buying a valuable gift for friend or for oneself). Participants read one positive and one negative outcome for each option, which were identified as equally likely and ordered from emotionally the most positive to the most negative for the protagonist. Participants were then asked which decision should be made so that the protagonist would avoid regret, no matter how the decision turned out.

Given the emotional ranking of possible outcomes, a decision that would ensure the avoidance of regret is the option *not* associated with the most negative outcome. When the most negative outcome was associated with the undesired option (e.g., studying for the exam but feeling left out from one's friends), a large majority of participants anticipated and avoided regret by choosing the desired option (e.g., going to a movie with friends). But when the most negative outcome was associated with a desired option (e.g., buying a valuable gift for oneself but disappointing a friend with no gift), significantly fewer college students and young adolescents avoided anticipated regret by choosing the undesired option. The young adolescents and college students were no different in their judgments, demonstrating the general influence of beliefs and desires on participants' ability to make decisions that anticipate and avoid regret.

Prior to being given the protagonists' rankings and making a decision, participants were asked to complete three component skills necessary to create the rankings and make a final regret-based decision. These skills included: a) generating possible positive and negative outcomes associated with each decision option; b) anticipating one's own feelings associated with each possibility being realized; and c) rank ordering those outcomes in light of anticipated feelings. In each case, the young adolescent group performed less methodically, less systematically, and in a more biased manner than the college students. Compared to the college students, the young adolescents generated fewer negative potential outcomes for desired options, anticipated the negative outcomes to desired options to be less affectively negative, and were more biased in more negatively rank ordering undesired than desired outcomes. The college students showed some, but substantially less, influence than the young adolescents of the desirability of options on their component abilities to anticipate and avoid regret.

The challenge in hypothetically thinking about regret goes beyond initially experiencing or anticipating regret to managing or regulating the emotion (Zeelenberg & Pieters, 2007). Generally speaking, once initiated, regret can be difficult to turn off, even if one wants to, and can lead to negative outcomes. Unregulated regret is related to insomnia (Schmidt & Van der Linden, 2009), general distress (Roese, Epstude, Fessel, Morrison,

Smallman, Summerville, et al., 2009), and poor coping after the end of a relationship (Saffrey & Ehrenberg, 2007).

The regulatory challenge posed by hypothetical thinking is sometimes so profound as to cause distress. A colleague who teaches *Psychology of Women and Gender* requires an assignment in which students are asked to imagine that they are gay and write a letter coming out to their parents. A week before the assignment was due, the professor received the following e-mail from a student in the class:

> As I read through the assignment and saw what it entails I began to feel very uncomfortable. I'm sorry but I truly cannot write these letters, thus I cannot do this assignment. It goes against everything inside of me. I understand that it is just an assignment, but to me it is more than that. By doing it I would have to put myself in that position by turning my thoughts to it, which will contradict everything I have been taught: that I believe. I do not want to put these thoughts in my mind for any reason.

Personal beliefs and values not only can *bias* hypothetical thinking – they can *stop* it cold! This student is not alone in being unwilling to entertain hypothetical possibilities because they conflicted with closely held beliefs and values. Politicians refuse to answer hypothetical questions all the time in fear of revealing their closely held values and beliefs (Kensley, 2003). Perhaps it is not surprising that such refusals occur when one is asked to think hypothetically about emotionally or politically salient issues. But the evidence suggests that hypothetical thinking is biased even in relatively cold emotional contexts. Kuhn, Amsel, & O'Loughlin (1988) demonstrated that adolescents and adults were biased when evaluating evidence for variables about which they held prior beliefs. In this research, participants reviewed a series of instances of potential causal variables associated with a positive or negative outcome. Two variables, one believed causal and one noncausal, were consistently associated with the positive outcome, suggesting that either one or both together could be causally related to the outcome.

Participants were to treat each variable as a possible cause of the outcome and test each against the data. But instead of treating variables *as if* they were possible causes, some participants just reiterated their beliefs that the variables were causal or noncausal. This failure to adopt a hypothetical attitude toward the variables was reflected in *belief-based* responses that melded theory and evidence into a single representation of "the way things are." Belief-based responses decreased in frequency from childhood to adulthood, but sporadic use of them remained prevalent among most adults. In other studies presented by Kuhn et al. (1988), participants were posed different forms of the test question to better clarify that prior beliefs were to be ignored and the variables treated as causal hypotheses. Although the procedure worked to reduce the prevalence of belief-based responses, it did not eliminate them, and age-related differences remained. Another way found to reduce belief-based responses was to use task content (laundry task versus plant task), which elicited less strongly held prior beliefs. But participants still used available beliefs to respond to questions in a belief-based manner.

Even when a hypothetical attitude toward the variables was adopted and participants evaluated variables against the data, prior beliefs undermined an objective and systematic evaluation of the evidence. Notably, the indeterminacy of the evidence was ignored, and "evidence-based" responses were made in a biased manner, with the same patterns of data being interpreted differently for variables believed to be causal and noncausal. There were very few cases of identical evaluations of the causal status of the pair of variables receiving the same pattern of evidence even among adult groups.

Subsequent research over the past twenty years has thoroughly tested the Kuhn et al.'s (1988) account of the development of skills to coordinate theory and evidence (see Lehrer & Schauble, 2006; Zimmerman, 2000, 2007). One line of research has identified skills to *implicitly* evaluate and revise beliefs about multicausal variables being acquired in childhood (e.g., Schulz & Bonawitz, 2007; Schultz, Gopnik, & Gilmore, 2007). These accounts of multicausal inferences do not require conscious reflection on and coordination of hypothetical beliefs and evidence. The findings do not deny the importance of *explicit* theory-evidence coordination, which may be necessary to articulately defend judgments to others or oneself (Kuhn & Dean, 2004).

Although not all evidence evaluation tasks require explicit theory-evidence coordination, performance on tasks that do demonstrates age/education- and task-related variability (Lehrer & Schauble, 2006; Zimmerman, 2000, 2007). For example, Amsel & Brock (1996) minimized task demands compared to Kuhn et al. (1988) by presenting participants with multiple pieces of evidence for a single variable paired with an outcome. Instances of healthy or sick plants were associated with the presence or absence of a causal (sun) or noncausal (charm) variable. Children, adolescents, non-college-educated adults, and college students held strong prior beliefs about the variables, which received the same patterns of evidence, so that variables believed causal and noncausal were both confirmed and disconfirmed. At each age group, participants additionally

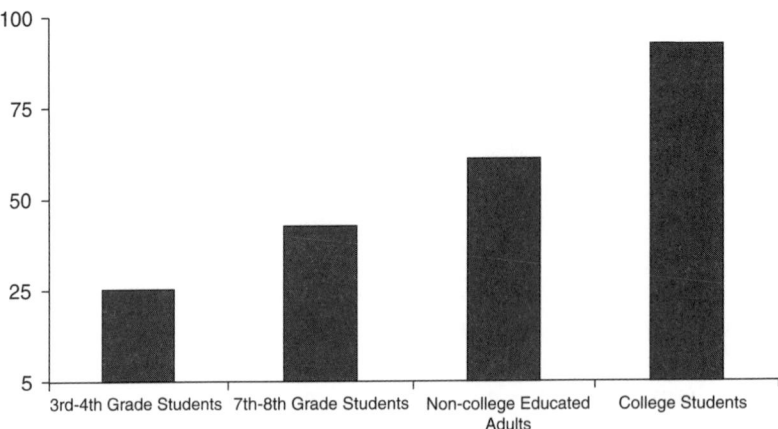

FIGURE 5.2. Percentage of evidence-based responses by age group in Amsel and Brock (1996).

were randomly assigned to conditions that presented the same instances of evidence for variables as the standard control group, but also included missing instances of data with either the status of the variable missing, the status of the outcome missing, or both missing. After all the instances in a trial were reviewed, participants rated their certainty of the causal status of the variable on a seven-point scale (from very certain the variable is causal to very certain the variable is noncausal) and justified those judgments.

Two key results are relevant here. First, even the youngest children in the study were responsive to the evidence, despite holding contrary beliefs for some variables. The ratings of each age group suggest that they distinguished the patterns of data, confirming their sensitivity to the evidence. This sensitivity to the evidence was further demonstrated by participants' ratings of the causal or noncausal status of variables in the presence of instances of missing data. Causal certainty ratings in these conditions were the same as (adult and college groups) or lower than (children and adolescent groups) the control condition that contained no missing data instances. The findings suggest that missing data were not treated as opportunities to project prior beliefs onto incomplete data, as would be expected if participants were merely using their prior beliefs to interpret the data.

Second, all participants' judgments and justifications were affected by their prior beliefs. There was a linear increase by age and education in justifying causal judgments by referring to the evidence (see Figure 5.2), replicating Kuhn et al. (1988). Also, all groups of participants differentially rated the causal status of variables believed causal and noncausal, despite the variables having been presented with the same evidence. The effect of prior beliefs on causal ratings was weakest among the college students and similar for the children, adolescents, and adults.

Hypothetical thinking skills underlie the ability to anticipate and regulate regret and to consciously entertain causal hypotheses and coordinate them with evidence. The skills involve the objective and systematic creation and evaluation of possible worlds and the interpretation of the real world in light of them. Armed with the ability to do so, reality is understood in light of possibilities, or as Piaget and Inhelder put it, reality becomes subordinated to possibilities. However, adults' processes of hypothetical thinking on these tasks are often subject to the biasing intrusions of real-world beliefs, knowledge, values, and desires that reflect a challenge in exercising the regulation necessary to ensure that hypothetical thinking is objective and systematic. Although the regulatory skills improve with age and education, even college students are challenged by the regulatory demands of hypothetical thinking.

DUAL PROCESS THEORY AND HYPOTHETICAL THINKING: THEORY AND APPLICATIONS

The same regulatory demands are echoed in the reviews of children's, adolescents', and adults' difficulties in reasoning about alternative possible worlds. The failure of children to critically reflect on alternative worlds was identified as the challenge limiting their ability to distinguish impossible from improbable events, to reason counterfactually, and to experience regret. Although adolescents and adults could reflect on alternative possible worlds, they had difficulties regulating the intrusion of real-world beliefs, knowledge, values, and desires into the process of creating, evaluating, and interpreting reality in light of possibilities. As a result, they had difficulty objectively and systematically anticipating and regulating regret and entertaining and evaluating causal hypotheses. The developmental trajectories for performance on all these tasks are different, but each has a common metacognitive challenge underlying the ability to objectively and systematically reason hypothetically.

In the present section, a dual process account of the hypothetical thinking is presented which proposes that the same metacognitive challenge underlies the ability to objectively and systematically think hypothetically. The metacognitive challenge involves consciously regulating cognitive processes so that a variety of hypothetical thinking skills can be coordinated in the service of interpreting the real world in light of alternative possible worlds. It is argued that the development of such metacognitive skills emerges in adolescence.

Dual process theory proposes the existence of two parallel cognitive systems: experiential and analytic. Experiential processing is regarded as the default processing system, responses from which are automatically activated and readily available. Such processing relies on concrete and contextualized task representations, rich in content from the situation, prior knowledge, beliefs, experiences, emotional reactions, and/or associations, often resulting in heuristic responding (Evans, 2006, 2007; Stanovich & West, 2000). Analytic processing is more conscious, effortful, and slower, often requiring the inhibition of experiential-based responses prior to the expression of analytic ones. Analytic processing may involve constructing decontextualized task representations that require knowledge and skills that are acquired in culturally specific contexts (e.g., schools), and resulting in responses that are normatively justified by formal logic or mathematics (Evans, 2006, 2007; Stanovich &West, 2000).

Evans (2006, 2007) provides a dual process account of hypothetical thinking on hypothesis-testing situations, including the theory-evidence coordination tasks reviewed here. One such assumption is that causal hypotheses are processed analytically as *epistemic* mental models that encode people's degree of belief, confidence, or uncertainty. So although processed differently than one's beliefs and knowledge regarding a particular variable, hypotheses are not held as epistemically neutral propositions (variable X is assumed to be neither causal nor noncausal), but as ones with epistemic status (e.g., variable X is assumed to have a low likelihood of being causal). Children who provide belief-based responses are likely not even engaging in analytic processing of variables as hypotheses, relying instead on experiential processing of their beliefs and knowledge that are automatically activated in the context. This does not mean that children do not revise beliefs in light of evidence, only that they do not consciously and effortfully reflect on the variables as hypotheses.

Adolescents, adults, and college students readily engage in the analytic processing of variables as hypotheses in hypothesis-testing contexts, as reflected by their rate of evidence-based responses. Nonetheless, they can still be influenced by the epistemic values associated with different hypotheses. As a given hypothesis is further assumed to be evaluated singularly and relative to its epistemic value (Evans, 2006, 2007), a causal hypothesis will be retained until evidence clearly requires its rejection. As a result, variables believed to be causal and noncausal may well be evaluated differently despite the presentation of the same evidence. From this perspective, adolescents, adults, and college students are not *motivated* to seek out confirming evidence, but rather they are consistent in testing hypotheses for which they have different degrees of credulity. Perhaps differences in evaluation for different hypotheses given the same evidence would disappear if participants were trained to adopt a general intellectual value that identical evidence must be interpreted identically for the different variables. Such may have been the case with advanced graduate students in Kuhn et al. (1988), who performed without bias on the theory-evidence coordination task.

The central assumption of Evans's (2006, 2007) dual process theory of hypothesis testing is the notion that to entertain and test hypotheses, default and automatic experiential processes must be inhibited in favor of conscious and effortful analytical processing. This regulation of the cognitive system to permit analytic processing of alternative possible worlds seems to be implicated in all other tasks considered in this review: modal reasoning, reasoning logically about possible (not pretend) worlds, counterfactual reasoning, and the regulation of regret. Children appear to have general difficulty doing this except in relatively restrictive contexts and with a good deal of support. However, adolescents and adults appear to do so spontaneously, but they may not always regulate their experientially based belief, knowledge, and desires carefully enough so they do not influence analytic reasoning processes.

In a recent line of research, I have been exploring the development of metacognitive skills to regulate dual cognitive processes (Amsel, Close, Sadler, & Klaczynski, 2009; Amsel, Klaczynski, Johnston, Bench, Close, Sadler, & Walker, 2008). The dual analytic and experiential processing systems need to be regulated so that the response associated with the more appropriate processing system would be expressed in the appropriate context. For example, probability judgments are made every day, and in many contexts a quick, experientially based heuristic estimate of the probability of events is sufficient to achieve a goal or complete a task. At other times, probability judgments require more serious and analytically based reflective, thoughtful, and mathematically sound analysis of the situation. Metacognitive skills are required to permit default experientially based responses to take precedence in the former case and analytically based responses in the latter case.

In a total of 5 studies involving more than 1,200 participants, we found that most preadolescents had notably poor metacognitive skills, failing to fully distinguish between analytical- and experiential-based responses. With age and education, most participants demonstrated a competent metacognitive status and correctly distinguished analytical- and experiential-based responses. Participants' metacognitive status predicted their performance on the ratio-bias task, in which they were presented with two equal gambles (e.g., 1/10 versus 10/100). Participants were told that the gambles were equivalent and asked if they had *no preference* between the gambles or a preference for one gamble or the other. A large majority of participants with a poor metacognitive status had a preference for one or the other gamble (typically the one with more absolute winners, 10/100), and some were even willing to pay for the preferred gamble. Most (although not all) participants with competent metacognitive status gave *no preference* responses, were almost never willing to pay for a preferred gamble, and actually gambled less than others. One notable finding (Amsel et al., 2008, Study 1) was that performance on the ratio bias task was better predicted by metacognitive status, which indexes regulatory ability, than by Mathematics ACT scores, which index analytic mathematical ability.

These findings identify the development of competencies to regulate dual analytic and experiential processes, deemed necessary for objective and systematic hypothetical thinking. Amsel et al. (2008, Study 3) point to the importance of metacognitive status for hypothetical thinking. Participants were asked to complete the same ratio-bias task and were randomly assigned to do so from their own perspective or that of a logical person. According to dual process theory of hypothetical thinking, the perspective instructions should elicit analytic processing to represent oneself *as if* one were a logical person, which should also result in more analytically based *no preference* responses on the ratio-bias task. That was exactly what happened. The data suggested that the manipulation improved the analytic responding and did so particularly for those who had some competence to distinguish between the dual processes.

Similar hypothetical thinking effects of improving reasoning on other tasks were realized by inviting participants to adopt the perspective of others. Using the insight from dual process theory, I explored whether Introductory Psychology students would score higher on a questionnaire assessing scientific beliefs about psychology when they were invited to think like their psychology professors (Amsel, Johnston, Alvarado, Kettering, Rankin, & Ward, 2009). We found that when Introductory Psychology students adopted the perspective of their Psychology professor, they affirmed the scientific basis of the discipline more strongly than they normally do, and affirmed those beliefs as strongly as senior psychology majors (Amsel, Baird, & Ashley, 2011). Performance on simple physics problems also improved when physics students were invited to think like their physics professors rather than as they normally do (Amsel & Johnston, 2008).

Inviting students to engage in hypothetical thinking about their professor's perspective on a discipline appears to help them think more analytically about the discipline and its assumptions. Future research is exploring the development of such hypothetical reasoning effects across a variety of different disciplines that make up the general educational curriculum of many universities (English, History, and Human Development).

SUMMARY AND CONCLUSIONS

The precise emergence of hypothetical thinking is difficult to pinpoint. However, it is reasonable to identify adolescence as the approximate time of emergence of hypothetical thinking for three reasons. First, there is a convergence of evidence from a range of tasks that specifically require reasoning about possible worlds that the ability to do so develops in later childhood or early adolescence. These tasks include treating alternative event sequences as possibilities, logically inferring consequences from possible worlds, counterfactual reasoning, experiencing or anticipating regret, and modal reasoning. Second, these tasks have in common a set of skills typically thought to be related to general cognitive and metacognitive development during adolescence (Kuhn, 2009). These skills include critical reflection (on possible worlds), systematic inferences (about those worlds), and objective interpretations (of reality in light of them). Third, there are critical metacognitive skills acquired during adolescence to regulate the dual processes and specifically to distinguish experiential and analytic processes (Amsel et al., 2008, 2009). Such skills are central to thinking analytically about possible worlds in the form of epistemic mental models and interpreting reality in light of them.

Armed with these general cognitive and metacognitive and specific hypothetical thinking skills, adolescents can interpret reality in light of possibilities, thereby achieving what Inhelder and Piaget (1958) proposed to be uniquely acquired by and transformative for adolescents: subordinating reality to possibilities. However, there remain many cases where adolescents and adults fail to reason hypothetically in an objective and systematic manner because of the influence of prior beliefs, knowledge, and desires. This was exemplified in hypothesis-testing research. However, such cases of bias were not motivated but can be traced to the inevitable consequence of analytically processing possible worlds as epistemic mental models. People may hold different epistemic values for the same possible worlds, and so may make different inferences about them and differently interpret reality in light of them. Even still, there remains the influence of experiential processes in analytic ones on a variety of hypothetical thinking tasks. Perhaps skills to reason hypothetically are subject to expertise effects. Adolescents may be novices at hypothetical thinking and become more objective and systematic in their hypothetical thinking through feedback and practice. For example, perhaps the negative consequences of experiencing *unanticipated* regret may make adolescents more motivated to think hypothetically and make decisions that anticipate and avoid regret.

Although the proposed model of hypothetical thinking is consistent with Piaget's claim about *when* hypothetical thinking is acquired, it is not consistent with *how* it is acquired. From the dual processing framework, hypothetical thinking is acquired in adolescence due to the development of general cognitive and metacognitive and specific hypothetical thinking skills but not the acquisition of formal logico-mathematical structures. Rather than holding that the development of hypothetical thinking is a by-product of formal logical ability indexed by combinatorial reasoning, the evidence suggests that it is a by-product of coordinating specific hypothetical reasoning skills to critically reflect on possible worlds and the metacognitive and regulatory skills to create, make inferences about, and interpret reality in light of possible worlds.

There is an ironic quip that goes, "Imagine a world without hypothetical thinking." It is hard to imagine such a world as the ability to think hypothetically is ubiquitous, representing some of the most fundamental and uniquely human forms of thinking. In an important way, the acquisition of hypothetical thinking makes adolescents adult-like. Although novices at it, hypothetical thinking is a transformative ability, enabling adolescents to understand reality in light of possibilities. There are documented ways in which hypothetical thinking, and the regulation of analytic and experiential processes it entails, affects the quality of judgments, reasoning, emotions, decision making, and learning. To perfect these skills, adolescents need practice in thinking hypothetically, which seems to be something they readily do.

REFERENCES

Albertson, K., & Shore, C. (2008). Holding in mind conflicting information: Pretending, working memory, and executive control. *Journal of Cognition and Development, 9*, 390–410.

Amsel, E., Baird, T., & Ashley, A. (2011). Misconceptions and conceptual change in undergraduate students' understanding of psychology as a science. *Psychology Learning and Teaching, 10*, 3–10.

Amsel, E., Bobadilla, W., Coch, D., & Remy, R. (1996). Young children's memory for the true and pretend identities of objects used in object-substitution pretense. *Developmental Psychology, 32*, 479–491.

Amsel, E., & Brock, S. (1996). The development of evidence evaluation skills. *Cognitive Development, 11*, 523–550.

Amsel, E., Close, J., Sadler, E., & Klaczynski, P. (2009). Awareness and irrationality: College students' awareness of their irrational judgments on gambling tasks. *The Journal of Psychology, 143*, 293–317.

Amsel, E., Cottrell, J., Sullivan, J., & Bowden, T. (2005). Anticipating and avoiding regret as a model of adolescent decision-making. In J. Jacobs & P. Klaczynski, (Eds.) *The development of judgment and decision-making in children and adolescence* (pp. 119–154). Mahwah, NJ: Erlbaum.

Amsel, E., & Johnston, A. (2008). *The role of imagination in conceptual change.* Paper presented at the Annual Meeting of AERA, March, New York, NY.

Amsel, E., Johnston, A., Alvarado, E., Kettering, J., Rankin, R., & Ward, M. (2009). The effect of perspective on misconceptions in psychology: A test of conceptual change theory. *The Journal of Instructional Psychology, 36*, 289–295.

Amsel, E., Klaczynski, P. A., Johnston, A., Bench, S., Close, J., Sadler, E., & Walker, R. (2008). A dual-process account of the development of scientific reasoning: The nature and development of metacognitive intercession skills. *Cognitive Development, 23*, 452–471.

Amsel, E., & Smalley, J. (2000). Beyond really and truly: Children's counterfactual thinking about pretend and possible worlds. In K. Riggs & P. Mitchell (Eds.), *Children's reasoning and the mind* (pp. 99–134). Brighton: Psychology Press.

Amsel, E., Trionfi, G., & Campbell, R. (2005). Reasoning about make-believe and hypothetical suppositions: Towards a theory of belief-contravening reasoning. *Cognitive Development, 20*, 545–575.

Beck, S. R., & Crilly, M. (2009). Is understanding regret dependent on developments in counterfactual thinking? *British Journal of Developmental Psychology, 27*, 505–510.

Beck. S. R., Robinson, E. J., Carroll, D. J., & Apperly, I. A. (2006). Children's thinking about counterfactuals and future hypotheticals as possibilities. *Child Development, 77*, 413–426.

Bourchier, A., & Davis, A. (2002). Children's understanding of the pretence-reality distinction: A review of current theory and evidence. *Developmental Science, 5*, 397–413.

Broughton, J. (1983). The cognitive developmental theory of adolescent self and identity. In B. Lee & G. Noam (Eds.), *Developmental approaches to the self.* New York: Plenum.

Carruthers, P. (2002). Human creativity: Its evolution, its cognitive basis, and its connections with childhood pretence, *British Journal for the Philosophy of Science, 53*, 1–25.

Dias, M. G., & Harris, P. J. (1988). The effect of make-believe play on deductive reasoning. *British Journal of Developmental Psychology, 6*, 207–221.

(1990). The influence of the imagination on reasoning in young children. *British Journal of Developmental Psychology, 8*, 305–318.

Dimant, R. J., & Bearison, D. J. (1991). Development of formal reasoning during successive peer interactions. *Developmental Psychology, 27*, 277–284.

English, L. D. (1993). Children's strategies in solving two- and three-dimensional combinatorial problems. *Journal for Research in Mathematics Education, 24,* 255–273.

Erikson, E. H. (1968). *Identity, youth and crisis.* New York: Norton.

Evans, J. St. B. T. (2006). The heuristic-analytic theory of reasoning: Extension and evaluation. *Psychonomic Bulletin and Review, 13,* 378–395.

(2007). *Hypothetical thinking: Dual processes in reasoning and judgment.* New York: The Psychology Press.

Fischbein, E., & Gazit, A. (1988). Combinatorial problem solving capacity of children. *Z.D.M. International Reviews on Mathematical Education, 5,* 1–12.

Friedman, O., & Leslie, A. M. (2007). The conceptual underpinnings of pretense: Pretending is not 'behaving-as-if'. *Cognition, 105,* 103–124.

Gallagher, J. M., & Reid, D. K. (1981). *The learning theory of Piaget and Inhelder.* Monterey, CA: Brooks/Cole.

Gilovich, T., & Medvec, V. (1995). The experience of regret: What, when, and why. *Psychological Review, 102,* 379–395.

Grinder, R. (1969). The concept of adolescence in the genetic psychology of G. Stanley Hall. *Child Development, 40,* 355–369.

Guajardo, N. R., Parker, J., & Turley-Ames, K. J. (2009). Associations among false belief understanding, counterfactual reasoning, and executive function. *The British Journal of Developmental Psychology, 27,* 681–702.

Guttentag, R., & Ferrell, J. (2004). Reality compared with its alternatives: Age differences in judgments of regret and relief. *Developmental Psychology, 40,* 764 –775.

(2008). Children's understanding of anticipatory regret and disappointment. *Cognition and Emotion, 22,* 815–832.

Harris, P. L. (2000). *The work of the imagination.* Oxford: Blackwell.

Harris, P. L., & Kavanaugh, R. D. (1993). Young children's understanding of pretense. *Monographs of the Society for Research in Child Development, 58 (1, Serial No. 231).*

Harris, P. L., German, T., & Mills, P. (1996). Children's use of counterfactual thinking in causal reasoning. *Cognition, 61,* 233–259.

Inhelder, I., & Piaget, J. (1958). *The growth of logical thinking.* New York: Basic Books.

Kahneman, D., & Tversky, A. (1982). The simulation heuristic. In D. Kahneman, P. Slovic, & A. Tversky (Eds.), *Judgment under uncertainty: Heuristics and biases* (pp. 201–208). New York: Cambridge University Press.

Kinsley, M. (2003). Just supposin': In defense of hypothetical questions. *Slate.* Accessed January 10, 2010 at http://www.slate.com/id/2089163

Kohlberg, L. (1984). *The psychology of moral development.* San Francisco: Harper & Row.

Kuhn, D., Amsel, E., & O'Loughlin, M. (1988). *The development of scientific thinking skills.* Orlando, FL: Academic Press.

Kuhn, D. (2001). How do people know? *Psychological Science, 12,* 1–8.

(2009). Adolescent thinking. In R.M. Lerner & L. Steinberg (Eds.), *Handbook of adolescent psychology,* (3rd ed., pp. 152–186). New York: John Wiley & Sons.

Kuhn, D., & Dean, Jr., D. (2004). Connecting scientific reasoning and causal infer-
ence. *Journal of Cognition and Development, 5,* 261–288.
Landsman, J. (1993). *Regret: Persistence of the possible.* New York: Oxford University
Press.
Lehrer, R., & Schauble, L. (2006). Scientific thinking and science literacy. In W.
Damon, R. Lerner, K. A. Renninger, & I. E. Sigel (Eds.), *Handbook of child psy-
chology: Child psychology in practice* (6th ed., Vol. 4, pp. 153–196). Hoboken,
NJ: John Wiley & Sons.
Leslie, A. M. (1987). Pretense and representation: The origins of "theory of mind".
Psychological Review, 94, 412–426.
Lillard, A.S. (2001). Pretend play as Twin Earth: A social-cognitive analysis.
Developmental Review, 21, 495–531.
Markovits, H., & Vachon, R. (1989). Reasoning with contrary-to-fact propositions.
Journal of Experimental Child Psychology, 47, 398–412.
McCloy, R., & Strange, P. (2009). Children's understanding of counterfactual
alternatives. In N. A. Taatgen & H. van Rijn (Eds.), *Proceedings of the 31th
Annual Conference of the Cognitive Science Society* (pp. 1627–1632). Austin, TX:
Cognitive Science Society.
Moshman, D. (1998). Cognitive development beyond childhood. In W. Damon
(Series Ed.) & D. Kuhn & R. Siegler (Vol. Eds.), *Handbook of child psychology:
Vol. 2. Cognition, perception, and language, 5th ed., (pp. 947–978).* New York:
Wiley.
   (2005). *Adolescent psychological development: Rationality, morality, and identity*
(2nd edition). Mahwah, NJ: Erlbaum.
Mueller, U., Sokol, B., & Overton, W. F. (1999). Developmental sequences in
class reasoning and propositional reasoning. *Journal of Experimental Child
Psychology, 74,* 69–106.
Nichols, S., & Stich, S. (2000). A cognitive theory of pretense. *Cognition, 74,*
115–147.
Perner, J. (1991). *Understanding the representational mind.* Cambridge, MA: MIT
Press.
   (2000). About + belief + counterfactual. In P. Mitchell and K. Riggs (Eds.),
Children's reasoning and the mind (pp. 367–401). New York: Psychology Press.
Perner, J., Baker, S., & Hutton, D. (1994). Prelief: The conceptual origins of belief
and pretence. In C. Lewis and P. Mitchell (Eds.), *Children's early understanding
of mind: Origins and development.* Hove: Erlbaum.
Piaget, J. (1962). *Play, dreams, and imitation in childhood.* New York: W.W. Norton
& Co.
   (1972). Intellectual evolution from adolescence to adulthood. *Human
Development, 15,* 1–12.
   (1987). *Possibility and necessity* (Vols. 1 and 2). Minneapolis: University of
Minnesota Press.
Rafetseder, E., Cristi-Vargas, R., & Perner, J. (2010). Counterfactual reasoning: Developing a sense of "nearest possible world". *Child Development, 81,*
376–389.
Rescher, N. (1961). Belief-contravening suppositions. *Philosophic Review, 70,*
176–195.

(1964). *Hypothetical reasoning*. Amsterdam: North-Holland Publishing.

Richards, C. A., & Sanderson, J. A. (1999). The role of imagination in facilitating deductive reasoning in 2-, 3- and 4-year-olds. *Cognition, 72*, 1–9.

Riggs, K. J., & Peterson, D. M. (2000). Counterfactual thinking in pre-school children: Mental state and causal inference. In P. Mitchell & K. J. Riggs (Eds.), *Children's reasoning and the mind* (pp. 87–99). Hove: Psychology Press.

Riggs, K. J., Peterson, D. M., Robinson, E. J., & Mitchell, P. (1998). Are errors in false belief tasks symptomatic of a broader difficulty with counterfactuality? *Cognitive Development, 13*, 73–90.

Robarge, J., & Flexer, B. (1979). Further examinations of formal operational reasoning abilities. *Child Development, 50*, 478–484.

(1980). Control of variables and propositional reasoning in early adolescence. *The Journal of Genetic Psychology, 103*, 3–12.

Robinson, E. J., & Beck, S. (2000). What is difficult about counterfactual reasoning? In P. Mitchell & K. J. Riggs (Eds.), *Children's reasoning and the mind* (pp. 101–119). New York: Psychology Press.

Roese, N., Epstude, K., Fessel, F., Morrison, M., Smallman, R., Summerville, A., et al. (2009). Repetitive regret, depression, and anxiety: Findings from a nationally representative survey. *Journal of Social & Clinical Psychology, 28*, 671–688.

Ruffman, T., Perner, J., Olson, D. R., & Doherty, M. (1993). Reflecting on scientifc thinking: Children's understanding of the hypothesis-evidence relation. *Child Development, 64*, 1617–1636.

Saffrey, C., & Ehrenberg, M. (2007). When thinking hurts: Attachment, rumination, and post-relationship adjustment. *Personal Relationships, 14*, 351–368.

Schmidt, R., & Van der Linden, M. (2009). The aftermath of rash action: Sleep-interfering counterfactual thoughts and emotions. *Emotion, 9*, 549–553.

Schulz, L. E., & Baraff-Bonawitz, E. (2007). Serious fun: Preschoolers engage in more exploratory play when evidence is confounded. *Developmental Psychology, 43*, 1045–1049.

Schulz, L. E., Gopnik, A., & Glymour, C. (2007). Preschool children learn about causal structure from conditional interventions. *Developmental Science, 10*, 322–332.

Selman, R. (1980). *The growth of interpersonal understanding*. New York: Academic Press.

Shtulman, A. (2009). The development of possibility judgment within and across domains. *Cognitve Development, 24*, 293–309.

Shtulman, A., & Carey, S. (2007). Improbable or impossible? How children reason about the possibility of extraordinary events. *Child Development, 78*, 1015–1032.

Skolnick, D., & Bloom, P. (2006). What does Batman think about SpongeBob? Children's understanding of the fantasy/fantasy distinction. *Cognition, 101*, 9–18.

Stanovich, K. E., & West, R. F. (2000). Individual differences in reasoning: Implications for the rationality debate. *Behavioral and Brain Sciences, 23*, 645–726.

Weisberg, D. S., & Bloom, P. (2009). Young children separate multiple pretend worlds. *Developmental Science, 12*, 699–705.

White, H. (1985). Breakdowns in combinatorial reasoning: The role of memory. *Journal of Genetic Psychology, 146,* 431–432.

Woolley, J. D. (1995). The fictional mind: Young children's understanding of pretense, imagination and dreams. *Developmental Review, 15,* 172–211.

(1997). Thinking about fantasy: Are children fundamentally different thinkers and believers from adults? *Child Development, 68,* 991–1011.

Wyman, E., Rakoczy, H., & Tomasello, M. (2009). Young children understand multiple pretend identities in their object play. *British Journal of Developmental Psychology, 27,* 385–404.

Zeelenberg, M., & Pieters, R. (2007). A theory of regret regulation 1.0. *Journal of Consumer Psychology, 17,* 3–18.

Zimmerman, C. (2000). The development of scientific reasoning skills. *Developmental Review, 20,* 99–149.

Zimmerman, C. (2007). The development of scientific thinking skills in elementary and middle school. *Developmental Review, 27,* 172–223.

PART II

SOCIAL AND CONTEXTUAL PERSPECTIVE

6

Testing, Testing: Everyday Storytelling and the Construction of Adolescent Identity

AVRIL THORNE AND LAUREN A. SHAPIRO

University of California, Santa Cruz

In the sixty years since Erik Erikson (1950) cast adolescence as the prime era for identity exploration, ample research has found that reflecting on who one is indeed accelerates with approaching adulthood (see reviews by Côté, 2009; Waterman, 1982). This development usually has been captured with questions repeatedly posed across several years' time that ask adolescents the degree to which they have struggled with and committed to a sense of who they are (see Côté, 2009; Schwartz, 2001). Consistent with the work of Erikson, these longitudinal surveys construe identity development as a self-reflective project that has little connection with the *immediate* social environment. Consequently, although much has been learned about the individual development of identity, the process through which identity develops in particular social contexts has remained elusive (Côté, 2009; Grotevant, 1987, 1997; Kroger, 1993; Penuel & Wertsch, 1995; Thorne, 2000, 2004).

The present chapter aims to complement this distal view of identity development by embedding the identity-making process in the everyday contexts in which adolescents make sense of their lives. Building on the work of Piaget, we suggest that the process by which adolescents reflect on their identities is empowered by their capacity for hypothetical thinking (Piaget, 1965; Piaget & Inhelder, 1969). However, we propose that hypothetical thinking is not just a thought experiment but also a social experiment that recruits the assistance of particular listeners. Overall, we view identity as continually constructed and reconstructed in the process of narrating emotional experiences to others with the aim of testing the congruence of one's own perspective with that of a valued listener. We construe this process as rife with developmental risk and opportunity. But we are getting ahead of ourselves.

We begin with the question of why identity is an important problem for adolescents, particularly in the context of western industrialized societies.

We next examine why stories are useful structures for making sense of lived experience. We then pursue storytelling as an active, collaborative process that engages the hearts and minds of both teller and listener, thereby exposing the elusive dynamics of self or identity development.[1] Finally, because systematic studies of in-situ storytelling have been rare with adolescents, we use case examples to suggest how adolescents learn who they are in the process of storying their experience to family members and friends. We conclude by considering what is gained and what is lost in construing adolescent identity development as a socially distributed process.

WHY IDENTITY IS AN IMPORTANT PROBLEM FOR ADOLESCENTS

According to Piaget, adolescence marks the advent of formal operations, the capacity to think in the abstract, to reason about that which is not immediately present, and to form and test theories (Inhelder & Piaget, 1958). At the core of the Piagetian tradition is the belief that human cognitive development is propelled forward through hypothesis testing. Advancing Piagetian theory beyond reasoning about the physical world, Harter (1999) suggested that adolescents apply their newly acquired cognitive abilities to the self. According to Harter, the self can be viewed as a theory, something that in its most perfect form is both testable and consistent. In adolescence, however, the self may feel anything but that.

Identity is perhaps most easily defined by its lack, a sense of uncertainty about who one is and what one wants and values (Erikson, 1968; Kroger, 2007). In western societies, there is ample reason for confusion on the part of adolescents and young adults because youth are generally allowed considerable choice with regard to their associates and activities (Arnett, 2000). The uncertainty is also biological because adolescents are beginning to inhabit a body that is radically different from the one they previously owned, perhaps causing them to question who they really are. For example, changes in hormone levels can trigger dramatic mood swings that can color one's feelings about oneself and others (Archibald, Graber, & Brooks-Gunn, 2007; Larson, Csikszentmihalyi, & Graef, 1980).

Adolescents also experience important changes in the quality and quantity of their roles and relationships. In white, middle-class families, adolescence ushers in a shift in relations between parents and children, which

---

[1] The disciplinary roots of the concepts of self and identity differ, with "self" being more social-psychological and "identity" being more age-developmental; however, the concepts increasingly merge in literature on adolescent and adult development (Côté, 2009).

tend to become increasingly egalitarian, with more equal give and take (Grotevant & Cooper, 1998). Another key development in adolescence is that social networks expand as youth explore new reference groups beyond the family of origin and transition to new schools (Reiss, Azmitia, Syed, Radmacher, & Gills, 2009). Recent work on identity development has emphasized the challenges that youth encounter as they navigate across different social worlds, such as from parents to peers and from home to school (Cooper, Domingues, & Rosas, 2005).

Fortunately, adolescents tend to become increasingly well equipped to make sense of themselves across these multiplying life domains. Mid-adolescents are especially prone to be troubled by whether they are truly being themselves, and whether they act the same from one setting to the next (Harter & Mansour, 1992). Their perceptions of self-worth tend to differ depending on the relationship context; for example, they tend to feel like a different person with parents than with teachers, and with male peers than with female peers (Harter, Waters, & Whitesell, 1998). Concern with self-consistency may be enhanced by the realization that one is known only superficially in one context (such as with a new friend) and more thoroughly in others (such as with family and with old friends). For older adolescents and young adults, transitions between different reference groups may become more comfortable as prior identifications, such as feelings about parents, are reformulated in light of current identifications with one's social and ideological worlds (Schachter, 2004).

Adolescents tend to become increasingly skilled at logical reasoning (Kuhn, 2009) and at making causal and thematic connections across the events of their lives (Habermas & de Silveira, 2008). With this growing capacity to synthesize different and sometimes contradictory events comes an alertness to incongruities between past and present selves and the ability to imagine different hopes and fears for the future. This cognitive development may allow identities to emerge that reconfigure multiple or conflicting senses of self (Erikson, 1950; Habermas & Bluck, 2000; Markus & Nurius, 1986; McAdams, 1985; Schachter 2004). In the next section, we consider how storytelling is implicated in generating, testing, and reflecting on hypotheses about the self.

STORIES AS EXQUISITE VEHICLES FOR MAKING SENSE OF LIVED EXPERIENCE

Human experience is incredibly rich, and stories select and filter experience by highlighting particular settings, characters, actions, and outcomes

(Labov & Waletzky, 1967; McAdams, 1993). This selection process is important because what gets storied is more likely to be remembered than what does not (Mandler & Johnson, 1977). Highly emotional experiences tend to disrupt expectations and to be especially prone to be remembered and storied (Brewer, 1988). Furthermore, highly emotional experiences, such as falling in love, learning to drive a car, or losing a loved one, are especially rife in adolescence and young adulthood, which tends to be the most memorable era of the lifespan (Robinson, 1992; Rubin, Rahhal, & Poon, 1998).

Our primary interest in highly emotional experiences, however, is not so much their superior memorability, but rather the process by which such events are evaluated. A crucial feature of a story is its meaning (Labov & Waletzky, 1967). Meaning is the subjective evaluation of why something happened or why it matters, the "point" of the story. The point of a story is often framed in terms of the needs or intentions of particular characters. Attributions of intentionality are so prevalent that such attributions have even been found in accounts of swirling triangles, whose motion is attributed to one triangle "trying to "chase" the others (Heider & Simmel, 1944). Explicit intentions or evaluations are especially likely to be constructed for events that are troubling because trouble demands an explanation (Bruner, 1990). For example, a serious argument with a friend is more likely to be accompanied by an explanation than is a story of a romantic evening (McLean & Thorne, 2003; Thorne, McLean, & Lawrence, 2004).

Individuals make meaning of a past experience through the filter of their ongoing experience. From a Jamesian (1890) perspective, this entails the currently experiencing "I" evaluating a "me" and potentially reconfiguring the meaning of that "me" in light of current concerns. In this way, personal storytelling entails time travel and perspective taking, seeing oneself in the past from the perspective of the present. Such time travel has been found to accelerate across adolescence, producing increasingly dense temporal, causal, and thematic connections or meanings across salient self-defining memories (e.g., Habermas & Bluck, 2000; Habermas & de Silveira, 2008; McLean, Pasupathi, & Pals, 2007).

The meanings that one makes of past experience are not necessarily peculiar to the teller but draw from larger systems of meaning, such as dominant cultural values or master narratives (Bamberg, 1997; Mishler, 1995). Master narratives are culturally prevalent messages or ideologies that regulate the social and emotional life of communities. For example, some master narratives dictate different emotional concerns for boys and girls ("big boys don't cry;" "good girls help others"; Brown & Tappan, 2008). Such master narratives have been observed in parent-child co-reminiscence as well as in the traumatic memory narratives of late adolescents (Fivush, 1991; Fivush et al., 2000; Thorne & McLean, 2002; Thorne & McLean, 2003). The latter studies found that a large proportion of traumatic memory narratives violated the tough-boy and caring-girl master narratives by expressing raw vulnerability in the face of trauma. For example, young men and women were equally likely to portray the death of a loved one as a poignant, painful experience rather than something that they had mastered by being stoic or concerned about the feelings of others who were also grieving (Thorne & McLean, 2003). Although we have barely begun to understand why particular master narratives may or may not be operative in particular settings, it is clear that the concerns of immediate listeners, such as a tenderhearted peer versus a stoic father, are an important factor (Thorne & McLean, 2003). We now turn to storytelling and identity making as a collaboration by considering how listeners help shape what people share about their lives and what it means.

STORYTELLING AS A COLLABORATIVE AND POTENTIALLY CONTENTIOUS PROCESS

Storytelling is not a reflex that emerges independently when the child begins to talk; rather, storytelling is a skill that is learned with the help of elders. Notably, parents of very young children initially choose the experiences that get storied. For example, a parent might ask "What happened when we went to the zoo today?" and may persist in asking the question until the child settles on the event that the parent wants to talk about, such as seeing a giraffe (Fivush & Nelson, 2006). Within a few years, children tend to learn to select and narrate events independently.

In addition to learning to narrate what happened, children also learn to narrate the emotional meaning of the event. By about age four, children in western cultures learn that perspectives on the emotional meaning of their experience may differ. For example, a parent may say "Remember when we went on that bike trip and you got so tired?" to which the child responds "I didn't get tired!" In expressing the emotional meaning of such experiences, the child comes to see that she can have a unique perspective on a shared past event (Fivush & Nelson, 2006). Parent-child talk about emotionally negative events, such as sadness, is especially critical for the development of an emotional self-concept (Fivush, Berlin, Sales, Mennuti-Washburn, & Cassidy, 2003). Negative emotions are particularly likely to be regulated by parents because anger, fear, and sadness can be burdensome for the family. Co-reminiscing about negative experiences teaches children how they should and should not represent their feelings to others.

In western societies, parental scaffolding of the child's narration of the past soon gives way to a more equal give and take. Longitudinal studies have found considerable support for collaborative "spiraling" during parent-child reminiscing, in which the adult and child increasingly come to embellish each other's perspectives (Fivush, Haden, & Reese, 1996). Whereas scaffolding is a pedagogical activity that teaches the child how to tell a story, spiraling is more socio-emotional, a sharing of experiences with the child in order to elaborate and negotiate their meaning. Negotiating the meaning of past experiences seems a more suitable representation of what transpires once a child has mastered the rudiments of storytelling. However, scaffolding may be applicable to what happens when novices of any age make sense of new experiences to listeners who are more competent in that domain.

Regardless of whether storytelling involves negotiating or scaffolding, an act of storytelling is generally a delicate maneuver. Stories that are told in everyday life are more likely to be ill-formed than stories that are written down or well rehearsed. The rough-hewn nature of everyday stories reflects the fact that such stories tend to be about new events whose meaning must be constructed (Thorne, Korobov, & Morgan, 2007), and because storytelling requires the cooperation of the listener. Even the process of launching a story is perilous because a story cannot be told without the support of the listener (Ochs & Capps, 2001). For example, a corpus of stories that spontaneously emerged in conversations between college-age friends contained plenty of instances in which stories were capsized or derailed (Thorne et al., 2007). For instance, in the following excerpt, Sue makes a bid to tell a story by introducing a topic that has a time-mark: "I got this ride from this freshman girl the other day. She was so funny." Her friend Amy abruptly interrupts the flow of the story by asking what the driver said. The interruption gets Sue off track and Amy then seizes the floor to tell her own story:

> SUE: I get this girl, I got this ride from this freshman girl the other day. She was so funny.
> AMY: *What'd she say?*
> SUE: What?
> AMY: What'd she say?
> SUE: I don't know. She was like talking about Santa Cruz. How much she loved it.
> And ... I don't know. It was just funny.
> AMY: Hmm. I always ... like when I went and picked up Marty ... And I was like, "You know I'm just going down to like Safeway or whatever," and he was like, "You know that's cool." [Amy's story continues]

A general principle of storytelling is that listeners tend to highlight information that unifies the action and thereby conveys the point of the story (van den Broek et al., 2003). However, the point of the story is not given in the event itself but is negotiated between teller and listener. In the preceding example, Amy pushed for a point that is not what Sue intended. Listeners have their own agendas and may look beyond the story to ask the teller "Why are you telling *me* this story? Why is it relevant to me?" For example, a girl who is telling a story about a bike might be asked "Do you think I'm going to buy you a bike?" (van den Broek et al., 2003). As a consequence of the different agendas that may emerge between teller and listener, storytelling sessions tend to be particularly rife with evaluations or feedback about the meaning of one's experience (Edwards & Middleton, 1988). Furthermore, because listener feedback of any sort tends to enhance the personal memorability of the event (Pasupathi, Stallworth, & Murdoch, 1998), social storytelling (versus, e.g., writing in a journal) may be an especially implicated in the formation of an identity.

Even with a cooperative listener, telling a story to someone else is considerably more complicated than telling a story to oneself because the teller must triangulate the meaning for the character in the story (the "me" for first-person stories), the meaning for the experiencing "I" who is telling the story, and the meaning for the listener (Bamberg, 1997). The listener's feedback may be overt or subtle, but even overt feedback can have mixed meanings. For example, in the following excerpt, John criticizes Phil's girlfriend for an insensitive remark. Phil tries to minimize the import of the remark, and John ultimately says she's a nice girl. But does John really mean it? And what meaning does Phil draw from the story?

> JOHN: and [your girlfriend] said that one time when we were all in the hall talking she said 'that's why I don't date popular guys' or something. *That was like fucked up (laughter) dude,* I was like whaat? (laughter) I was like man, I was like "that's not cool" and you were like "psh, whatever like whatever." I was like "well you should probably let him go to some parties" and then like
>
> PHIL: yeah
>
> JOHN: and like (laughter) I don't know
>
> PHIL: *yeah I don't know she makes a lot of cracks like that, but she's joking so*
>
> JOHN: yeah
>
> PHIL: *that's cool though*
>
> JOHN: *she, I don't know seems like a nice girl though. Like she's fun to talk to and stuff.*

In the preceding excerpt, John seems to invoke a master narrative that girlfriends should not publicly criticize their boyfriends. Phil casts the criticism as a joke, implying that John does not know Phil's girlfriend as well as Phil does. Phil then seems to invoke a counternarrative, that a friend should not criticize one's girlfriend. This episode nicely illustrates that storytellers invoke more than their own and the listener's perspective because such perspectives draw from more general networks of cultural ideologies that regulate social, emotional, and moral life (Bamberg, 2004). Interest in such ideologies blossoms in adolescence with the development of the capacity for hypothetical thinking and helps propel the development of life stories and identity (Hankiss, 1981; McAdams, 1985).

To date, research on the development of ideologies in adolescents' life stories has been distal rather than proximal; that is, ideologies have been examined in life-story monologues collected across several years' time, but not in dialogues (Habermas & Bluck, 2000; Habermas & de Silveira, 2008). Attending to patterns of ideological positioning that develop through life-story dialogues is an important frontier for understanding the process of adolescent identity development (Bamberg, 2004; Davies & Harré, 1990; Talbot, Bibace, Bokhour, & Bamberg, 1996; Thorne & McLean, 2003).

The notion of master narrative positioning brings serious business to everyday storytelling, the business of navigating diverse and potentially conflicting cultural assumptions and ideologies (Bamberg, 1997; Mishler, 1995; Turiel, 2003), any number of which potentially can be invoked in the course of an exchange about "what does this really mean?" Whereas master narratives presumably preexist in the cultural consciousness, master narrative positioning takes place in the here and now. In the process of exchanging personal stories, tellers and listeners are at each other's mercy with regard to which master narratives to invoke, resist, or transform. We now look specifically at the kinds of identity testing that emerge as adolescents story their experiences to others.

VIGNETTES OF HOW ADOLESCENT IDENTITIES GET TESTED IN THE PROCESS OF EVERYDAY STORYTELLING

As previously noted, research with adolescents rarely has examined how identities get tested through storytelling. However, a classic study by Grotevant and Cooper (1985) comes close. Grotevant and Cooper (1985) observed the kinds of family interactions that differentiated adolescents assessed as generally high or low on level of identity exploration. Family interactions were observed in the context of planning a hypothetical family vacation. Adolescents who showed high levels of identity exploration were especially likely to experience a family rhetoric of mutuality that not only supported but also challenged the adolescent's individuation from other family members. That is, families who both agreed and disagreed, and who compromised and restated each other's feelings encouraged adolescent identity exploration.

Because the Grotevant and Cooper's (1985) study remains one of the few systematic examinations of adolescent identity exploration in the context of conversations in close relationships (see also Hauser, Allen, & Golden, 2006), it is instructive to consider how their findings might be applicable to reminiscing about the past instead of planning the future. Planning and reminiscing are similar in that both social activities entail the expression and coordination of multiple points of view. However, as previously noted, acts of reminiscing are particularly prone to concern highly emotional experiences (Brewer, 1988). For this reason, we expect that reminiscing is especially saturated with emotional framing and reframing, and that listener support and challenges to the emotional meaning of a reminiscence are a particularly potent force in identity making.

The following excerpt illustrates some of the challenges that can occur when adolescents and other family members engage in reminiscence. The excerpt is from a family dinner table conversation that we collected from three generations of Andersons. Ella, the target adolescent, is thirteen. Her grandmother is in her eighties and her uncle is in his sixties. We have highlighted some dynamics in italics:

> UNCLE: Yeah, well mom and dad went off and took [oldest daughter] to Washington D.C. when we lived in Tennessee, I guess I was thirteen.
> GRANDMOTHER: Yeah, you were thirteen then.
> UNCLE: And I was thirteen and I took care of all three little kids. *Could you imagine that, Ella?*
> GRANDMOTHER: The youngest one was two-and-a-half.
> UNCLE: We went to get on the bus and go to downtown Knoxville, Tenessee.
> ELLA: *But weren't they babies?*
> GRANDMOTHER: *The two-and-a half-year-old could walk!*
> ELLA: *Wouldn't they get scared?*
> GRANDMOTHER: *Why should they be scared?*

In this episode, Ella is being pressed to take the perspective of her uncle, who was her age at the time (*Could you imagine that, Ella?*). Ella is game; she tries to imagine it and expresses concern that a thirteen-year-old was left with three "babies" in his care (*But weren't they babies?*). The grandmother challenges the characterization that she left her "babies" behind (*The two-and-a-half-year-old could walk!*). But Ella shifts the question to the emotions of the youngsters: *Wouldn't they get scared?* which the grandmother challenges, *"Why should they be scared?"*

Ella is both being tested by and is testing the elders' ideology with regard to the capabilities of a thirteen-year-old. The elders challenge her claim that a thirteen-year-old is not capable of being a responsible caregiver. Ella's response to this challenge nicely illustrates resistance to scaffolding. From an Eriksonian perspective (Schachter, 2004), Ella is being urged to reconfigure her childhood identifications, to shift her perspective with regard to how grown up a thirteen-year-old can and should be.[2]

Challenges to one's perspective about who one is and what one can do might be growth enhancing but might also be crippling. Because the meaning of feedback from listeners can take time to sink in, we have found it useful to collect retrospective accounts of salient episodes of memory telling, in which we ask for a story of what led one to tell the story, to whom, how the story was told, the listener's reaction, and one's own reaction (Thorne & McLean, 2003). Perhaps surprisingly, most of the late adolescents we have studied are able to recount salient episodes of memory telling, some in quite vivid detail, even though the memorable telling usually occurred some time ago. We have found that there is often a big time gap, averaging about three years, between the memorable event and the memorable telling, with an equivalent gap between the memorable telling and the point at which the memorable telling is reported, typically at age nineteen (Thorne & McLean, 2002). The fact that the memorable event, the memorable telling, and the reporting tend to span the entire range of adolescence suggests that a brief episode of telling one's past to others can be very salient (Thorne, 2000).

We have also found that narratives in which the listener did not embrace the storyteller's emotional perspective were usually more detailed and nuanced than narratives in which the listener was understanding and sympathetic (Thorne & McLean, 2003). Particularly poignant were narratives of listeners' responses to a disclosure of raw vulnerability or suffering. Nearly half of these vulnerability narratives fell on deaf ears. Listeners did not want to hear bad news, and/or they did not know what to do with it.

---

[2] Much more is going on in this episode than meets the eye. A stranger to this family would have little idea as to what underlies the grandmother's emphasis that Ella reframe what counts as "scary," or Ella's view that the babies should have been scared. We had special access to this family, a requisite for good narrative research (Eagan & Thorne, 2010).

Listeners' reactions can drive inward an experience that took considerable courage to disclose. Steve, for example, recounted an event from his junior year of high school in which he confessed to his girlfriend Kate his growing feelings of inferiority with regard to her and their friends:

> I felt inferior to her and to her relationships with two of our other friends. This inferiority complex pervaded every aspect of our relationship, and also every aspect of my own opinion of myself. Soon there wasn't a single thing I did that I didn't hate myself for doing, whether productive or not. I remember that, as these feelings were creeping up on me I tried to tell Kate, herself. I described terrible visions that my mind was forcing upon me and that I was afraid for my own sanity. All this frightened her. It did so much more harm than good that I now refrain from telling people about it in any more than vague terms.

Recalling this episode several years later, Steve continues to feel the force of inferiority on himself and others: "To this day I am cursed with a constant reaction of comparing: comparing myself unfavorably to others, comparing others unfavorably to others and comparing others unfavorably to myself. And I know it drives people away."

Disclosing vulnerabilities to friends can result in self-isolation as well as the contamination of the meaning of past and current relationships. For example, Kimberly recounted a childhood experience of being spanked by her father:

> When I was 8, I was playing with my Dad at some family friends' house and while he was talking to his buddy, I smacked him on the ass really hard and ran away giggling. As I was running upstairs, he grabbed me by the shirt and spanked me. I was surprised at his reaction.

Ten years later, Kimberly recounted telling this childhood event to her boyfriend:

> I was talking with my boyfriend about whether our parents ever hit or spanked us. I told him about this event. He wanted to know whether it made me scared of my Dad after that. I said it did and he was understanding. It made me reevaluate my feelings about my relationship with my Dad.

In this case, the listener endowed the event with more serious meaning than Kimberly intended, leading her to question the quality of her relationship with her father.

Listeners who respond to personal stories more seriously than was intended can also revive buried meanings for the teller. The backdrop of the following incident is that Carla essentially lost her father in childhood, when he became addicted to methamphetamines and took to life on the streets. In late adolescence, she was walking with a friend and suddenly caught sight of her father sitting on a bench:

> As we passed a bench I froze abruptly and gasped, my heart must have stopped. I thought I saw my father sitting there. We have not yet seen each other for years. I'm fairly positive it was him. My friend was confounded, she had never seen me react like that. The story just eased out of me, naturally as if a perfectly natural explanation for my behavior. She was pretty quiet and grave, and it made me realize that this memory which I've told to my closest friends had become almost a reflex story. I had numbed out to how traumatic and tragic the event was for me. Her reaction brought back the pain.

Of course, not all listeners are alike. A big problem in adolescence is finding the right audience to tell one's troubles to (Azmitia, Ittel, & Radmacher, 2005; Thorne & McLean, 2003). This search is exquisitely captured in the following narrative from Rachel, who recounted a horrific experience of being brutally raped at age fifteen and her ensuing search for the right listener:

> I have told boyfriends and close friends of mine what happened to me and they would all react differently. The *male friends* (*not boyfriends*) I told would get frustrated like they would have to console me and comfort me but they didn't know how to. Most of *my boyfriends* handled it with aggression (blamed the fact that I wouldn't have sex with them on the rapist). They went out and beat him up but that was the last thing I wanted. Recently I have told some *close girlfriends* of mine what happened and they have been very understanding. They cried with me and let me release the tension that I have been feeling for so long. They helped me realize that what happened was not my fault.

In the process of searching for the right audience, Rachel essentially discovered the force of gendered master narratives (Fivush et al., 2000). Male friends either did not know what to say or displayed aggressive self-interest – in both cases, the wrong response. Her close girlfriends gave her what she wanted, an openly sympathetic response.

Testing what can be told to whom establishes boundaries between the personal and the public self. Although this testing presumably occurs across much of the life course, adolescence is arguably dense with such experiments because one's reference groups are expanding at the same time that one begins to actively explore new forms of intimacy. As social networks expand, there is a high turnover in who knows what about one's life.

Compared to parent-child reminiscence, which has been studied primarily with regard to events that were mutually experienced (e.g., Fivush & Nelson, 2006), adolescents' stories of their past are more likely to be news to the listener. Deciding how much to tell in orienting a potential friend about one's past is not merely a question of efficiency; it is a matter of choice, based partly on one's assessment of what is gained by telling and what is risked. Furthermore, the disclosure that tends to occur between adolescent friends is a double-edged sword. Adolescent friends have more rights to each other's personal domain than do parents of adolescents (Smetana, Metzger, Gettman, & Campione-Barr, 2006) but are also more likely than parents to challenge meanings (Cooper & Cooper, 1992).

Trust in a potential audience can be brokered by a listener. Here is an excerpt from our corpus of conversations between close same-sex friends, college roommates whom we will call Irma and Elaine. Irma is gay and has a "thing" with Alice. Irma is generally closeted about her sexual orientation except with Elaine, who challenges Irma's secrecy in this episode:

ELAINE: You know the thing with you and Alice?
IRMA: What thing with me and Alice?
ELAINE: Well, you sort of have been secretive about your relationship.
IRMA: Oh oh yeah.
ELAINE: Mary [their roommate] was so upset about that 'cuz –
IRMA: She was upset because I didn't tell her?
ELAINE: Yeah, she's like "what I hate more is just like being left in the dark. I hate feeling like there's people are being secretive. I just want her to open up. I don't care what the issue is, I just want to know who this girl is that she brings home and what's going on with them."

Through this exchange, Irma learns that her secret is a burden to Elaine, who does not want to keep it and would prefer it be shared with others.

Testing who can be trusted with one's secrets can also entail testing whether it is okay to change who one is. In the following narrative, Omar describes what happened when he told his best friend Felicia why he kissed a boy:

I told my best friend Felicia, because I had to explain why I kissed a boy. I took her out for sushi the next day and told her how I felt. Her reaction wasn't too great. She had felt that I had lied to her about my sexuality for two years. I was very confused and I didn't know what to say. It took a while but things have been resolved.

In this instance, being honest about his sexuality had the inadvertent effect of upsetting his friend, who felt betrayed. Felicia assumed that Omar's sexual orientation was a secret that he had been withholding, whereas Omar felt that his sexuality was something that he was still trying to figure out. The complexity of sexual orientation is particularly salient to the current generation of American adolescents, for whom gender and sexuality are less clear-cut and more multifaceted than in prior eras (Diamond, 1998).

The following episode also highlights the tension between self-consistency and change. At age eighteen, Laura experienced a personal triumph when she managed to climb to the top of a mountain in the Rockies, a feat that she felt made her more courageous and brave. Afterward, she called her boyfriend:

> I told him on the phone that night what I had done. I felt pretty excited but he didn't seem that happy for me because *he felt that whenever he tried to get me to do something hard, I couldn't do it, but in this case when I wasn't with him I could.* At the time I got kind of mad at his reaction, but now I am still proud of myself and his reaction doesn't bother me.

Whereas Laura's boyfriend tried to enforce her self-consistency, self-consistency can also be self-regulated through narrative activity. In the following episode, Melissa broadcasts widely her self-consistency as a very independent woman:

> I was standing in the "second grade line" in the field of my private elementary school. (We were required to stand in the field and recite the Pledge of Allegiance every day before classes started). My "boyfriend" at the time was standing behind me and some of our friends were singing that children's song **** and **** are sitting in a tree, k-i-s-s-i-n-g … I got really upset at my "boyfriend" and told him that he wasn't allowed to tell anyone that we liked each other. This memory often comes up when I'm trying to explain to someone how I've ALWAYS been someone who doesn't like to be defined as a "girlfriend" in a relationship. I am a person who gets really crowded in a relationship and I tend to push people away on a regular basis. We (my friends and I) usually just laugh about my memory – saying "It all started when I was just a second-grader."

We do not know whether Melissa can maintain this ideology of self-consistency indefinitely, but if she changes, she will have to account for that change to herself and to her friends, perhaps altering, in the process, the meaning of the second-grade memory.

Overall, these narratives suggest that in the expanding social world of adolescents, the act of telling one's past to others is rife with risk and opportunity. With the capacity to test the boundaries between the public and the personal self and between personal sameness and change comes a vulnerability to being shaped by listeners' reactions. For better or for worse, telling one's past can simultaneously restructure one's sense of who one is, one's relationship with other characters in the story, and with the listener.

META-THEORETICAL ISSUES WITH REGARD TO LOCALIZING IDENTITY WORK IN EVERYDAY STORYTELLING

During the last decade, our interest in embedding identity work in the proximal social contexts in which adolescents story their lives has been met with several notable objections on the part of colleagues in developmental and personality psychology. One concern is that everyday storytelling is too fleeting. It has also been argued that construing the teller as being shaped by the listener compromises an agentic view of development. Other researchers have asserted that we are promoting a view of multiple identities as opposed to a coherent unified identity. Finally, our work has been criticized as overly encapsulated in a western view of adolescence. We will briefly consider each of these issues in turn.

With regard to the first concern, an act of storytelling is indeed fleeting. However, the fact that salient emotional experiences can be remembered for many years suggests that a single moment can be a meaningful touchstone to which one returns again and again. A momentary past experience not only can extend through time; it also can extend through social space because telling experiences to others distributes one's own life into the life of the community. As noted by Bruner (1990, p. 138), "Selves are not isolated nuclei of consciousness locked in the head, but are distributed interpersonally." Telling a past event can be so vivid as to revive the original experience not only for the teller, but also for a listener who was not present at the original event (Brewer, 1988). In short, an act of storytelling can extend through vast expanses of time and space, and this expansion is importantly implicated in the meaning of the story and the meaning of one's identity.

A second concern is that by construing the teller as being at the mercy of the listener we compromise an agentic view of development. From our perspective, the view that individuals are agents of their own development is overly romantic and as extravagant as the view that individuals are pawns of their environments. The perception that one is controlled by others is only possible because of an awareness that the opposite is also possible, that one can control others' reactions. Another way of framing what happens during moments of personal memory telling and thereafter is that tellers can choose to surrender or to resist the listener's apparent meaning. In short, the agency lies not only in the collaboration but also in the consequences for the narrative once feedback is implicitly or explicitly offered.[3]

With regard to the third concern, the issue of multiple identities versus a single unifying identity, we take a mid-way position between advocating for a highly local multiplicity (e.g., Bamberg, 2004) and for a highly trans-temporal and trans-spatial unified identity (e.g., Erikson, 1950; McAdams, 2001). In support of a view of local multiplicity, personal stories told in everyday life do show considerable change with regard to what is told and to whom (McAdams et al., 2006; Thorne, Cutting, & Skaw, 1998), and spontaneous storytelling between friends shows considerable variety in story content even across a ten-minute time span (Thorne, Korobov, & Morgan, 2007). However, while sympathetic to the notion of complicated and perhaps kaleidoscopic identities (Deaux & Perkins, 2001), we suggest that multiple identities are anchored and shaped by the weight of one's own past and the expectations of self and significant others (see also Thorne, 2004). The press for continuity may be particularly true in western societies, which tend to emphasize the value of self-consistency (Suh, 2002). If the western ideology of self-consistency is indeed so potent, multiple selves would seem especially difficult to maintain.

The fourth concern is a serious limitation: Our approach is definitely encapsulated in a western view of adolescence and, in particular, middle-class American society. Not only were we born and bred in this demographic, but all of the narrative examples in this chapter were collected from white and mostly middle-class American youth. Comparisons of parent-child storytelling in white middle-class American, working-class African-American, and Asian communities have revealed compelling differences with regard to storytelling practices and values (e.g., Miller, 1994; Miller & Sperry, 1988; Miller, Wiley, Fung, & Liang, 1997). To date, very little of this work has compared adolescent storytelling in different cultural communities. In addition, because adolescents increasingly inhabit a multicultural world, it is important to observe how adolescents from radically different cultural backgrounds reciprocally test the meaning of their own and each other's stories (Hammack, 2009).

---

[3] We thank Eric Amsel for helping us think through the issue of agency.

CONCLUSION

The search for identity often has been represented in the literature as how adolescents psychologically struggle with the question "Who am I?" Drawing from a Piagetian perspective, we view this struggle as an outgrowth of adolescents' growing cognitive capacity to experiment with and test self-meanings by sharing emotional experiences with others. Drawing from a Vygotskian perspective (Penuel & Wertsch, 1995), we view "Who am I" questions as internalizations of questions posed by others, such as "Who are you?" We have thus proposed that the quest for a sense of self or identity be addressed not as an individual phenomenon but as an everyday social pursuit. This pursuit creates special problems for adolescents because their intended audience is simultaneously expanding toward diverse reference groups and telescoping toward intimacy. In the process of proffering salient parts of one's past to a chosen audience, adolescents actively test the boundary between the public and personal self, and their sense of self as consistent and changing. It is here that we can most vividly see the pushes and pulls of past and present selves, for which personal storytelling is both rudder and sail.

ACKNOWLEDGMENTS

This work is based on the first author's plenary address to the annual meetings of the Jean Piaget Society, Quebec City, Canada, June, 2008. Funding was provided by NIH training grant T32 HD46423. Feedback from Eric Amsel, Judi Smetana, Margarita Azmitia, Paul Nelson, and Kelly Gola was very helpful as we revised this chapter.

REFERENCES

Archibald, A. B., Graber, J. A., & Brooks-Gunn, J. (2007). Pubertal processes and physiological growth in adolescence. In G. R. Adams & M. D. Berzonsky (Eds.). *Blackwell handbook of adolescence* (2nd Ed., pp. 24–47). Malden, MA: Blackwell Publishing.

Arnett, J. J. (2000). Emerging adulthood: A theory of development from the late teens through the twenties. *American Psychologist, 55*(5), 469–480.

Azmitia, M., Ittel, A., & Radmacher, K. (2005). Narratives of friendship and self in adolescence. In N. Way & J. V. Hamm (Eds.), The experience of close friendships in adolescence. *New Directions for Child and Adolescent Development, 107,* 23–39.

Bamberg, M.G.W. (1997). Positioning between structure and performance. *Journal of Narrative and Life History, 7*(1–4), 335–342.

(2004). "I know it may sound mean to say this, but we couldn't really care less about her anyway." Form and functions of "slut bashing" in male identity constructions in 15-year-olds. *Human Development, 47*, 331–353.

Brewer, W. F. (1988). Memory for randomly sampled autobiographical events. In U. Neisser & E. Winograd (Eds.), *Remembering reconsidered: Ecological and traditional approaches to the study of memory* (pp. 21–90). Cambridge: Cambridge University Press.

Brown, L. M., & Tappan, M. B. (2008). Fighting like a girl fighting like a guy: Gender, identity, ideology, and girls at early adolescence. In M. Azmitia, M. Syed, & K. A. Radmacher (Eds.), *The intersections of personal and social identities. New Directions for Child and Adolescent Development, 120*, 47–59.

Bruner, J. S. (1990). *Acts of meaning.* Cambridge, MA: Harvard University Press.

Cooper, C. R., & Cooper, R. G. (1992). Links between adolescents' relationships with their parents and peers: Models, evidence, and mechanisms. In R. D. Parke & G. W. Ladd (Eds.), *Family-peer relationships: Modes of linkages* (pp. 135–158). Hillsdale, NJ: Erlbaum.

Cooper, C. R., Dominguez, E., & Rosas, S. (2005). Soledad's dream: How immigrant children bridge their multiple worlds and build pathways to college. In C. R. Cooper, C. Garcia Coll, W. T. Bartko, H. Davis, & C. Chatman (Eds.), *Developmental pathways through middle childhood: Rethinking diversity and contexts as resources* (pp. 235–260). Mahwah, NJ: Erlbaum.

Côté, J. E. (2009). Identity formation and self-development in adolescence. In R. M. Lerner & L. Steinberg (Eds.), *Handbook of adolescent psychology* (Vol. 1, pp. 266–304). Hoboken, NJ: John Wiley & Sons.

Davies, B., & Harré, R. (1990). Positioning: The discursive production of selves. *Journal for the Theory of Social Behaviour, 20*, 43–63.

Deaux, K., & Perkins, T. S. (2001). The kaleidoscopic self. In C. Sedikides & M. B. Brewer (Eds.), *Individual self, relational self, collective self* (pp. 299–313). Philadelphia: Taylor & Francis.

Diamond, L. M. (1998). Development of sexual orientation among adolescent and young adult women. *Developmental Psychology, 34*, 1085–1095.

Eagan, J., & Thorne, A. (2010). Life stories of troubled youth: Meanings for a mentor and a scholarly stranger. In K. C. McLean & M. Pasupathi (Eds.), *Narrative development in adolescence: Creating the storied self* (pp. 113–130). New York: Springer.

Edwards, D., & Middleton, D. (1988). Conversational remembering and family relationships: How children learn to remember. *Journal of Social and Personal Relationships, 5*, 3–23.

Erikson, E. H. (1950). *Childhood and society.* New York: Norton.

(1968). *Identity: Youth and crisis.* New York: Norton.

Fivush, R. (1991). Gender and emotion in mother-child conversations about the past. *Journal of Narrative and Life History, 1*, 325–341.

Fivush, R., Berlin, L. J., Sales, J. M., Mennuti-Washburn, J., & Cassidy, J. (2003). Functions of parent-child reminiscing about emotionally negative events. *Memory, 11* (2), 179–192.

Fivush, R., Brotman, M., Buckner, J. P., & Goodman, S. H. (2000). Gender differences in parent child emotion narratives. *Sex Roles, 42*, 233–253.

Fivush, R., Haden, C., & Reese, E. (1996). Remembering, recounting, and reminiscing: The development of autobiographical memory in social context. In D. C. Rubin (Ed.), *Remembering our past: Studies in autobiographical memory* (pp. 341–383). Cambridge: Cambridge University Press.

Fivush, R, & Nelson, K. (2006). Parent-child reminiscing locates the self in the past. *British Journal of Developmental Psychology, 24,* 235–251.

Grotevant, H. D. (1987). Toward a process model of identity formation. *Journal of Adolescent Research, 2,* 203–222.

(1997). Identity processes: Integrating social psychological and developmental approaches. *Journal of Adolescent Research, 12,* 354–357.

Grotevant, H. D., & Cooper, C. R. (1985). Patterns of interaction in family relationships and the development of identity formation in adolescence. *Child Development, 56,* 415–428.

(1998). Individuality and connectedness in adolescent development: Review and prospects for research on identity, relationships, and context. In E. Skoe & A. von der Lippe (Eds.), *Personality development in adolescence: A cross national and lifespan perspective* (pp. 3–37). London: Routledge.

Habermas, T., & Bluck, S. (2000). Getting a life: The emergence of the life story in adolescence. *Psychological Bulletin, 126,* 248–269.

Habermas, T., & de Silveira, C. (2008). The development of global coherence in life narratives across adolescence: Temporal, causal, and thematic aspects. *Developmental Psychology, 44*(3), 707–721.

Hammack, P. L. (2009). Exploring the reproduction of conflict through narrative: Israeli youth motivated to participate in a coexistence program. *Peace and Conflict, 15,* 49–74.

Hankiss, A. (1981). Ontologies of the self: On the mythological rearranging of one's life history. In D. Bertaux (Ed.), *Biography and society: The life history approach in the social sciences* (pp. 203–209). Beverly Hills, CA: Sage Publications.

Harter, S. (1999). *The construction of the self: A developmental perspective.* New York: The Guilford Press.

Harter, S., & Monsour, A. (1992). Developmental analysis of conflict caused by opposing attributes in the adolescent self-portrait. *Developmental Psychology, 28*(2), 251–260.

Harter, S., Waters, P., & Whitesell, N. R. (1998). Relational self-worth: Differences in perceived worth as a person across interpersonal contexts among adolescents. *Child Development, 69* (3), 756–766.

Hauser, S. T., Allen, J. P., & Golden, E. (2006). *Out of the woods: Tales of resilient teens.* Cambridge, MA: Harvard University Press.

Heider, F., & Simmel, M. (1944). An experimental study of apparent behavior. *American Journal of Psychology, 57,* 243–259.

Inhelder, B., & Piaget, J. (1958). *The growth of logical thinking from childhood to adolescence.* New York: Basic Books.

James, W. (1890). *Principles of psychology* (Vol. 1). London: Macmillan.

Kroger, J. (1993). On the nature of structural transition in the identity formation process. In Kroger, J. (Ed.), *Discussions on ego identity.* Hillsdale, NJ: Lawrence Erlbaum Publishers.

(2007). *Identity development: Adolescence through adulthood.* Thousand Oaks, CA: Sage.

Kuhn, D. (2009). Adolescent thinking. In R. M. Lerner & L. Steinberg (Eds.), *Handbook of adolescent psychology* (Vol. 1, pp. 152–186). Hoboken, NJ: John Wiley & Sons.

Labov, W., & Waletzky, J. (1967). Narrative analysis. In J. Helm (Ed.), *Essays on the verbal and visual arts* (pp. 12–44). Seattle: University of Washington Press.

Larson, R., Csikszentmihalyi, M., & Graef, R. (1980). Mood variability and the psychosocial adjustment of adolescents. *Journal of Youth and Adolescence, 9,* 469–490.

Mandler, J. M., & Johnson, N. S. (1977). Remembrance of things parsed: Story structure and recall. *Cognitive Psychology, 9,* 111–151.

Markus, H., & Nurius, P. (1986). Possible selves. *American Psychologist, 41*(9), 954–969.

McAdams, D. P. (1985). *Power, intimacy, and the life story: Personological inquiries into identity.* Homewood, IL: Dorsey Press.

(1993). *The stories we live by: Personal myths and the making of the self.* New York: William Morrow.

(2001). The psychology of life stories. *Review of General Psychology, 5,* 100–122.

McAdams, D. P., Bauer, J. J., Sakeda, A. R., Anyidoho, N. A., Machado, M. A., Magrino-Failla, White, K. W., & Pals, J. L. (2006). Continuity and change in the life story: A longitudinal study of autobiographical memories in emerging adulthood. *Journal of Personality, 64* (5), 1371–1400.

McLean, K. C., Pasupathi, M., & Pals, J. L. (2007). Selves creating stories creating selves: A process model of narrative self-development in adolescence and adulthood. *Personality and Social Psychology Review, 11,* 262–278.

McLean, K. C., & Thorne, A. (2003). Adolescents' self-defining memories about relationships. *Developmental Psychology, 39,* 635–645.

Miller, P. J. (1994). Narrative practices: Their role in socialization and self-construction. In U. Neisser & R. Fivush (Eds.), *The remembering self: Construction and accuracy in the life narrative* (pp. 158–179). New York: Cambridge University Press.

Miller, P. J., & Sperry, L. L. (1988). Early talk about the past: The origins of conversational stories of personal experience. *Journal of Child Language, 15,* 293–315.

Miller, P. J., Wiley A. R., Fung, H., & Liang, C-H. (1997). Personal storytelling as a medium of socialization in Chinese and American families. *Child Development, 68*(3), 557–568.

Mishler, E. G. (1995). Models of narrative analysis: A typology. *Journal of Narrative and Life History, 5,* 87–123.

Ochs, E., & Capps, L. (2001). *Living narrative: Creating lives in everyday storytelling.* Cambridge, MA: Harvard University Press.

Pasupathi, M., Stallworth, L.M., & Murdoch, K. (1998). How what we tell becomes what we know: Listener effects on speakers' long-term memory for events. *Discourse Processes, 26,* 1–25.

Penuel, W. R., & Wertsch, J. V. (1995). Vygotsky and identity formation: A sociocultural approach. *Educational Psychologist, 30,* 83–92.

Piaget, J. (1965). *The moral judgment of the child.* New York: Free Press.

Piaget, J., & Inhelder, B. (1969). *The psychology of the child.* New York: Basic Books.

Reis, O., Azmitia, M., Syed, M., Radmacher, K., & Gills, J. (2009). Patterns of social support and mental health among ethnically-diverse adolescents during school transitions. *European Journal of Developmental Science, 3,* 39–50.

Robinson, J. A. (1992). First experience memories: Contexts and functions in personal histories. In M. A. Conway, D. C. Rubin, H. Spinnler, & W. A. Wagenaar (Eds.), *Theoretical perspectives on autobiographical memory* (pp. 223–239). Amsterdam: Kluwer Academic Publishers.

Rubin, D. C., Rahhal, T. A., & Poon, L. W. (1998). Things learned in early adulthood are remembered best. *Memory and Cognition, 26,* 3–19.

Schachter, E. P. (2004). Identity configurations: A new perspective on identity formation in contemporary society. *Journal of Personality, 72,* 167–200.

Schwartz, S. J. (2001). The evolution of Eriksonian and neo-Eriksonian identity theory and research: A review and integration. *Identity: An International Journal of Theory and Research, 1,* 7–58.

Smetana, J. G., Metzger, A., Gettman, D. C., & Campione-Barr, N. (2006). Disclosure and secrecy in adolescent-parent relationships. *Child Development, 77*(1), 201–217.

Suh, E. M. (2002). Culture, identity consistency, and subjective well-being. *Journal of Personality and Social Psychology, 83,* 1378–1391.

Talbot, J., Bibace, R., Bokhour, B., & Bamberg, M. (1996). Affirmation and resistance of dominant discourses: The rhetorical construction of pregnancy. *Journal of Narrative and Life History, 6,* 225–251.

Thorne, A. (2000). Personal memory telling and personality development. *Personality and Social Psychology Review, 4,* 45–56.

(2004). Putting the person into social identity. *Human Development, 47,* 361–365.

Thorne, A., Cutting, L., & Skaw, D. (1998). Young adults' relationship memories and the life story: Examples or essential landmarks? *Narrative Inquiry, 8,* 1–32.

Thorne, A., Korobov, N., & Morgan, E. (2007). Channeling identity: A study of storytelling in conversations between introverted and extraverted friends. *Journal of Research in Personality. 41,* 1008–1031.

Thorne, A., & McLean, K. C. (2002). Gendered reminiscence practices and self-definition in late adolescence. *Sex Roles, 46,* 267–277.

(2003). Telling traumatic events in adolescence: A study of master narrative positioning. In R. Fivush & C. Haden (Eds.), *Connecting culture and memory: The development of an autobiographical self* (pp. 169–185). Mahwah, NJ: Erlbaum.

Thorne, A., McLean, K. C., & Lawrence, A. M. (2004). When remembering is not enough: Reflecting on self-defining memories in late adolescence. *Journal of Personality, 72,* 513–541.

Thorne, A., & Nam, V. (2009). The storied construction of personality. In P. Corr & G. Matthews (Eds.), *Cambridge handbook of personality* (pp. 491–505). Cambridge: Cambridge University Press.

Turiel, E. (2003). Resistance and subversion in everyday life. *Journal of Moral Education, 32*(2), 115–130.

van den Broek, P., Lynch, J., & Naslund, J. (2003). The development of comprehension of main idea in narratives: Evidence from the selection of titles. *Journal of Educational Psychology, 95,* 707–718.

Waterman, A. L. (1982). Identity development from adolescence to adulthood: An extension of theory and a review of research. *Developmental Psychology, 18,* 341–358.

7

Adolescents' Social Reasoning and Relationships with Parents: Conflicts and Coordinations Within and Across Domains

JUDITH G. SMETANA

University of Rochester

The nature and quality of adolescents' relationships with parents is one of the most heavily researched topics in the study of adolescence (Smetana, Campione-Barr, & Metzger, 2006). In popular culture, there is a persistent perception that adolescence is a difficult period. Adolescents are thought to be selfish, preoccupied, and moody, and their relationships with their parents are said to involve generational strife, disrespect, and willful disobedience. Yet, overwhelming evidence from decades of psychological research indicates that extreme moodiness and alienation from parents, active rejection of adult values and authority, and youthful rebellion are the exception, not the norm. Only a small proportion of adolescents experience emotional turmoil and extremely conflicted relationships with parents. Those who do typically had problems and difficulties in their relationships with parents prior to adolescence (Collins & Laursen, 2004; Laursen & Collins, 2009; Smetana, 2011; Smetana et al., 2006). Moreover, high levels of conflict during adolescence clearly have negative consequences for adolescent development, relationships, and future adjustment (Laursen & Collins, 1994).

Although the storminess of the developmental period has been overemphasized, parent-child relationships do go through significant transformations during adolescence. Longitudinal studies indicate that adolescents' daily moods become increasingly negative in the transition to and during adolescence (Larson, Moneta, Richards, & Wilson, 2002; Larson & Richards, 1994). Among American ethnic minority and majority youth alike, feelings of support, closeness, and intimacy with parents decline, although there is some variation in when during adolescence this occurs (Fuligni, 1998; Furman & Buhrmester, 1985, 1992). Bickering, squabbling, and disagreements over everyday issues appear to be a normative feature of parent-adolescent relationships (Collins & Laursen, 2004; Holmbeck, 1996;

Smetana, 1996), not just in western cultures but worldwide (Smetana, 2011). According to a meta-analysis (Laursen, Coy, & Collins, 1998), conflicts with parents increase in frequency in early adolescence and then taper off; they increase in intensity from early to middle adolescence, leveling off after that. Indeed, moderate amounts of conflict during adolescence have been associated with better adjustment than either no conflict or frequent conflict (Adams & Laursen, 2001).

Why does conflict increase and closeness decline? Numerous explanations have been offered for these changes in parent-adolescent relationships, although most researchers believe that adolescent-parent conflict is a temporary perturbation that is adaptive for adolescent development (Holmbeck, 1996; Laursen & Collins, 2009). My research, discussed in this chapter, provides a social-cognitive and domain-specific perspective on these issues. My claim in this chapter is that focusing on coordinations in adolescents' social reasoning and understanding can illuminate some of the particular challenges of parent-adolescent relationships. In the next sections, I provide a brief overview of my findings on adolescents' and parents' reasoning about conflicts and their beliefs about the legitimacy of parental authority. Then, I discuss more recent research on adolescents' strategies and reasons for concealing information from parents. Finally, I discuss several explanations for these findings, including the role of peers, developmental changes in personal concepts, and cross-domain coordinations of personal, moral, and social concepts.

ADOLESCENTS' AND PARENTS' REASONING ABOUT CONFLICT

Adolescents' Perspectives on Conflict

The following two examples are drawn from interviews with European-American middle-class adolescents about their everyday conflicts with parents (Smetana, 1989). Although both examples pertain to conflicts regarding keeping the bedroom clean, adolescents' responses were fairly typical of the types of justifications adolescents gave for a variety of issues.

> TEEN: It is easier to throw things on the floor than hang them up or put them in my drawers.
> INTERVIEWER: Why do they want you to keep your room clean?
> TEEN: Well, my mother is one of those spotless people. She wants every-thing in perfectly neat order. That's it. I mean if it is not army-neat then forget it. I mean, I think it is good because it will teach me to clean up and

keep things clean. So my apartment, when I get older, doesn't look like a mess. But I should be able to live like I want to live.

INTERVIEWER: Why?

TEEN: Because it is my room and she doesn't live in there, I do. I'll close the door and not let anyone come in. It's not like it is dirty. It is just cluttered. It's not like I'm living with bugs and mice.

...

TEEN: At least in my room I'm sort of comfortable when it's messy. I'll clean it up, and it seems sort of cold. My parents would rather see it nice and neat. They'd rather see the rest of the house nice and neat, which I can appreciate, the rest of the house, but my room is my own.

INTERVIEWER: Why is it ok for you to do that?

TEEN: Because. My room is where I'm supposed to be ... it's sort of like my space, so I should be able to keep it the way I want to.

INTERVIEWER: So why do your parents think it is important to keep your room clean?

TEEN: They said it's dangerous in case of a fire, if you have garbage up there it rots, and you can get ants and stuff, but I don't keep any food up there. And it looks bad, but I don't take that many people up to my room anyway.

INTERVIEWER: Why do your parents think its wrong to leave it messy?

TEEN: Well, most people think that it's better to be neat than messy. It gives a better outward appearance. You know, if I came to school with my hair still the same way it was when I got up, that gives a certain image. But nobody really sees my room except my good friends, and they don't care. They know me anyway, so I don't mind.

Both of these early adolescents viewed their room as their private space. Therefore, they asserted that decisions about its condition should be up to them. As the second adolescent explained, parents have the legitimate authority to set standards regarding the rest of the house, but not regarding their room. Both teenagers view the condition of their room as a personal issue.

On the surface, these responses appear consistent with the popular view of adolescents as selfish, lazy, and disobedient. But recent theorizing and research from the framework of social domain theory (Nucci, 2001; Smetana, 1995, 2006, 2011; Turiel, 1983, 2002, 2006) suggest otherwise. In fact, adolescents' responses can be seen as reflecting a developmentally adaptive set of concerns. From the social domain perspective, this reasoning reflects adolescents' attempts to understand the self, construct an identity, and assert control over specific areas of their lives. Rather than reflecting defiance and resistance to parents' authority, these responses are part of a developmental and conceptual system of social knowledge that has been referred to as the *personal* domain. Personal issues pertain only to the actor and, as such, are judged to be beyond the bounds of social and moral regulation (Nucci, 1996, 2001, 2008; Smetana, 1995, 2006, 2011; Turiel, 1983, 2002, 2006). They are part of the private aspects of one's life and entail issues of preference and choice. Personal issues pertain to privacy, control over one's body, and choice and preferences. In the United States, these choices pertain to clothes, friends, and recreational activities. Nucci (1996, 2001) has claimed that although the content and breadth of the personal domain may vary across cultures, individuals in all cultures claim some issues as within their personal sphere. This is because claiming personal control over some issues is psychologically necessary to maintain a sense of agency, effectance, and uniqueness. In the context of conflict with parents, appeals to personal choice reflect adolescents' attempts to gain greater autonomy.

Adolescents' conflicts with parents are not just about the state of their bedrooms. They pertain to a range of issues, including doing chores, keeping the bedroom clean, choice of activities, doing homework, curfews, choice of friends, appearances, health and hygiene, and getting along with siblings. Although conflicts are over different issues, studies of European-American and African-American families (reviewed in Smetana, 2011) have shown that adolescents treat the majority of their conflicts as issues of personal choice or personal jurisdiction. In different studies, these justifications accounted for approximately half of adolescents' responses (with the remainder of responses spread among other categories, described in more detail later). Moreover, reflecting the expansion of the personal domain, adolescents' personal reasoning increased with age (Smetana, Daddis, & Chuang, 2003). And these responses were not restricted to youth growing up in cultures that are typically described as individualistic. Similar responses also have been obtained among Chinese adolescents residing in Hong Kong and China (Yau & Smetana, 1996, 2003), as well as among ethnic minority (African-American, Chinese, Latino, Filipino) youth in the United States (Fuligni, 1998; Smetana, Campione-Barr, & Daddis, 2004).

Parents' Perspectives on Conflict

Adolescents and parents generally agree on the issues (like the condition of adolescents' bedrooms) that cause conflicts in their relationships. But as the previous examples suggest, adolescents and parents have different interpretations of these issues. Whereas adolescents focus on the personal dimensions of their disputes, the preceding examples suggest that parents may have other concerns. Indeed, in individual interviews, parents expressed concerns with the perceived negative consequences of violating group norms ("What will Aunt Minnie think if she sees your room looking that way?"), maintaining social order ("your room is a mess – how can you find your stuff?"), coordinating the family social system ("everyone has their job, and if we all do them, things will work smoothly"), enforcing their authority ("It's my house, and I'm the boss"), and maintaining appropriate statuses and roles ("that's my job – that's what parents are supposed to do"). Parents also articulated the need for respect ("he shouldn't talk to his father like that"), appealed to familial and cultural norms ("that's the way we do it in this family"), and expressed the need for learning responsibility. All of these responses can be seen as pertaining to society, social organization, and *social conventions*.

According to social domain theory, these concerns form another system of social knowledge that is distinct from personal issues. Social conventions refer to the norms and regularities that promote the smooth and efficient functioning of social groups. Social conventions are defined as arbitrary, agreed-on, and shared regularities (like etiquette and manners) that coordinate the interactions of individuals within different social systems (Turiel, 1983, 2002, 2006). But not all regularities pertain to social conventions. Social conventions also have been differentiated from *moral* concepts. Moral concepts have been defined as prescriptive judgments regarding how individuals ought to behave toward each other. Whereas social conventions pertain to social organization and the social system, moral concepts pertain to justice, welfare, and rights. Moral concepts are generalizable across contexts and independent of particular rules or authority dictates. That is, they are wrong (or beneficial) because of their consequences for others' rights and welfare.

Across different studies, about half of parents' reasoning about conflicts pertained to social conventions, whereas moral reasoning accounted for only about 10–15 percent of responses (both among parents and teens). Consistent with the definition of the moral domain, moral conflicts generally focused on interpersonal relationships, such as how teens got along with their siblings. Parents were not only concerned with protecting teenagers from harm and with regulating social conventions; they also wanted to promote their flourishing. Parents' reasoning also included psychological justifications pertaining to the types of personality characteristics they hoped to instill (or that they found irritating). Parents also reasoned pragmatically, focusing on the practical importance for adolescents' future success of behaviors like doing homework and getting good grades.

Another prominent concern, as illustrated in adolescents' descriptions of parents' reasoning, was with teens' safety and health. Adolescents described their parents as worrying about "bugs and mice," that a mess was "dangerous in case of a fire," and that having "rotting garbage" means that "you can get ants and stuff." These concerns, along with others arising in arguments pertaining to issues such as bedtime ("she'll be tired tomorrow in school, and she needs to get her sleep"), curfew ("I need to know where he is and what he's doing, when he comes in late, I worry"), and choice of activities ("she doesn't realize what can happen in situations like that;" "playing video games is okay in moderation, just not eight hours a day. And they're probably bad on his eyes") have been referred to as *prudential* issues. Prudential issues pertain to individuals' comfort, health, safety, and harm to the self, and as the preceding examples suggest, these concerns also were prominent in parents' reasoning.

Conflict as (a Lack of) Interpersonal Coordination

As this suggests, adolescents and parents have different interpretations of the issues that cause conflict in their relationships. Adolescents claim personal jurisdiction over issues that parents view as social-conventional or prudential. And this is not just because adolescents and parents do not grasp the other's point of view. In our interviews, and in addition to providing justifications for their own perspectives, we also asked adolescents and parents to articulate the other's view on the disputes. As the examples at the outset of the chapter suggest, adolescents (and parents) accurately understood – but typically rejected – the other's perspectives.

Thus, one explanation for the increases in conflict during adolescence simply is that parents and adolescents are unable to coordinate their differing perspectives on disputes. This is because they have different stakes in the issues; their different goals lead them to view situations in different ways. Adolescents desire more autonomy and believe that they have the right to treat contested issues as personal. Parents, who view their role as protectors and socializers, are more likely to take a conservative stance and consider the conventional and prudential dimensions of issues. Although they endorse independence as an important developmental goal, they do not always agree that their adolescent has the developmental maturity and competence to exercise autonomy in particular situations.

HETEROGENEITY IN SOCIAL THOUGHT

Appeals to personal choice are not unique to adolescence. Consistent with the social domain view, there is compelling evidence that the personal domain emerges in early childhood. Social domain researchers claim that personal, conventional, and moral concepts reflect conceptually and developmentally distinct domains of social knowledge. They are distinct because they are constructed out of qualitatively different social interactions. And because social domain theory focuses on broad features of social interactions (like whether the interactions pertain to others' welfare or to choice), it is proposed that similar types of social interactions facilitate the development of knowledge in different social domains across different contexts and cultures. This does not preclude the finding of cultural differences (particularly in the form of cultural conventions and the boundaries and content of the personal domain). However, research has supported the proposition that different forms of social knowledge coexist within individuals and across cultures.

Research has shown that mothers' and children's social interactions around personal issues differ qualitatively from their interactions around moral and conventional issues. Unlike moral and conventional issues, which rarely involve compromise or concession, mothers of young children have ways of implicitly communicating to their children that personal issues can be negotiated. For instance, they offer choices ("do you want to wear the red sweater or the yellow one?" Nucci & Weber, 1995). Furthermore, interviews with European-American mothers of young children (Nucci & Smetana, 1996), as well as Japanese, Chinese, Brazilian, and African-American mothers (see Smetana, 2002, 2011 for reviews) indicate that mothers believe that granting children developmentally appropriate freedoms over a limited set of issues facilitates children's development. Thus, although mothers believe in the overall importance of fostering children's independence, they do not always agree about whether independence is appropriate or warranted in particular instances.

Most of the empirical work stemming from the social domain perspective has focused on children's and adolescents' ability to differentiate among (and coordinate between) different domains of social knowledge. A great deal of research, reviewed elsewhere (Smetana, 1995, 2006, 2011) has supported the claim that from early childhood on, children differentiate among moral, conventional, and personal issues, particularly when judging hypothetical situations that are considered prototypical of the domains. Personal understanding develops alongside an understanding of moral and social-conventional issues. This does not imply, however, that all events and social situations can be simply or cleanly separated into moral, conventional, or personal components. The social world is complex. Some events (particularly in real life) may be multifaceted and involve overlaps among the domains. In addition, the constructive nature of social development means that individuals may have different construals of particular situations. Individuals may apply concepts in different ways due to cultural and contextual differences, differences in their life circumstances, their informational assumptions (that is, their beliefs about the nature of reality), and the salience of different features of situations.

Beliefs about Legitimate Parental Authority

The research on adolescents' and parents' reasoning about conflict demonstrates that conflicts typically are about who has the right to control different issues. Parents and adolescents have different views of where to draw the line between parents' legitimate authority to make rules and regulate different types of issues and adolescents' desires for more control and personal freedom. But the studies of adolescent-parent conflict focus specifically on areas of disagreement. Studies of adolescents' and parents' beliefs about parents' legitimate parental authority to make rules about different types of issues (see Smetana, 2011 for a detailed review) reveal that along with disagreements, there also are substantial areas of agreement about what parents legitimately can control and what they cannot.

Our studies have shown that adolescents ranging from ten to eighteen years of age and their parents both strongly endorse parents' right to regulate moral, conventional, and prudential issues. They also believe (at least to varying degrees) that adolescents have the right to control personal issues. However, adolescents and parents disagree over where the boundary between parents' legitimate authority and adolescents' control over the self should be drawn. In the research on parental authority beliefs, this divergence was captured in a set of items referred to as multifaceted. Multifaceted issues (like cleaning the bedroom, getting a piercing, or hanging out with friends that parents dislike) are defined as issues that overlap the domains and that contain personal as well as conventional or prudential components. These items reflect the types of disagreements in perspectives that were evident in adolescents' and parents' reasoning about conflicts. And unlike straightforward moral, conventional, and prudential issues, there were significant discrepancies in adolescents' and parents' judgments of them. Parents viewed themselves as having a great deal more authority to control these issues than adolescents believed they did.

Moreover, there were age-related differences in judgments. Both cross-sectional and longitudinal studies confirmed that both adolescents' and parents' judgments of parents' legitimate authority declined dramatically across adolescence. These declines did not reflect a rejection of all parental authority; rather, they were domain-specific and reflected expansions in the boundaries of adolescents' personal domain. This was particularly evident in evaluations of multifaceted issues; there were parallel declines across adolescence in both parents' and adolescents' judgments of parents' authority to regulate these issues. We also observed longitudinal declines with age in African-American mothers' – but not adolescents' – judgments of their authority to make rules about personal issues (Smetana, Crean, & Campione-Barr, 2004). Furthermore, research among ethnic minority youth in the United States and elsewhere around the world has shown similar age-related increases in what adolescents consider to be under their personal jurisdiction (Cumsille, Darling, Flaherty, & Martinez, 2009; Darling, Cumsille, & Martinez, 2008; Fuligni, 1998; Smetana et al., 2004; Zhang & Fuligni, 2006). There are some individual differences in the patterning of this normative developmental trajectory that are associated with parenting (Cumsille, Darling, Flaherty, & Martinez, 2006; Cumsille et al., 2009), as well as a pattern of rejection of parental authority that appears to be associated with a trajectory of deviance and problem behavior. The overall trend, however, is toward age-related changes in the boundaries of parental authority.

It is important to note that this expansion consistently appears to come "from the bottom up." That is, at each age, adolescents claim more personal jurisdiction than parents allow. Adolescents push for more autonomy and parents gradually grant it. Thus, my claim is that adolescent-parent conflict, which reflects disagreements over the boundaries of parents' legitimate authority, provides one way of expanding those boundaries. It provides a context for negotiating autonomy and for transforming the nature of parent-adolescent relationships to allow greater adolescent independence and personal control.

Adolescents' Reasoning and Strategies for Information Management

Conflict is not the only way of obtaining autonomy, however. Across ages and among youth of different ethnicities and cultures, the majority of conflicts with parents typically are resolved by teens complying with their parents' demands (Smetana, 2011). Among European-American families, there is also a small but significant age-related increase in parents' concessions to teens' wishes. At least in my research, we have not seen this transfer of authority among families of other ethnicities or cultures, although Chinese adolescents in Hong Kong and China report a small but significant increase in compromise or joint resolutions (Yau & Smetana, 1996, 2003). Nevertheless, adolescents usually do what parents want them to do.

There is growing evidence, however, that middle adolescents increasingly adopt other strategies to short-circuit the negotiation process. This appears to be even more prevalent among youth who feel that they cannot express their disagreements overtly and therefore do not gain autonomy directly through negotiations over conflicts. As adolescents spend more time away from home and in the company of peers, they have more opportunities to conceal their activities from their parents. And it appears that they do. Recent evidence suggests that with age, adolescents increasingly manage the information they are willing to share with parents (Finkenauer, Engels, & Meuss, 2002; Keijsers et al., 2010; Keijsers, Frijns, Branje, & Meeus, 2009; Laird & Marrero, 2010; Smetana, Villalobos, Tasopoulos-Chan, Gettman, & Campione-Barr, 2009). Nondisclosure, topic avoidance, and secrecy increase in middle adolescence, just as the frequency of conflicts with parents declines and their intensity peaks.

Adolescents may decide not to share information about their activities with parents for a variety of reasons, and these reasons are linked with the types of activities they conceal. In our research, we have found that American adolescents do not disclose to parents about personal issues because they believe that their activities and feelings are private, personal, not harmful, and none of their parents' business (Smetana et al., 2009). In contrast, they do not tell their parents about their involvement in prudential issues of risk (like drinking alcohol, smoking cigarettes, and engaging in unprotected sex) primarily because parents would disapprove or they would get in trouble (Smetana et al., 2009; Smetana, Villalobos, Rogge, & Tasopoulos-Chan, 2010; Yau, Tasopoulos-Chan, & Smetana, 2009). And consistent with the definition of multifaceted issues as overlapping the domains, they do not disclose about multifaceted issues both because they fear parental disapproval or punishment and because they view these behaviors as personal and not harmful.

Although the patterns are similar for American youth of different ethnicities, there are some culturally distinctive patterns (Yau et al., 2009). Controlling for parental education and generational status, Chinese-American adolescents disclosed less to parents about personal activities, and particularly personal feelings, than Mexican-American and European-American youth did because they believed that their parents would not listen or understand. Mexican-American youth disclosed less to parents about prudential issues of risk (and were more involved in these risky behaviors) than did European-American teens because they were more concerned than other youth with parental disapproval and punishment.

European-American adolescents' reasons for not disclosing their activities to their parents also were associated with the strategies they used to manage this information (Smetana et al., 2009). When adolescents believed that their parents would disapprove of their behavior or that they would get in trouble, they either avoided discussing the issue or lied to parents. Lying was infrequent compared to other strategies for managing information. It was associated with more problem behavior, like drinking alcohol and experimenting with drugs, especially among middle adolescents as compared to early adolescents. However, lying became more normative with age. Middle adolescents lied more to parents than did early adolescents. Nearly a third of the tenth-graders who feared parental disapproval for their actions reported lying as their predominant strategy for managing information about risky prudential activities.

In contrast, adolescents rarely lied about personal activities, and when they did, they reported feeling more depressed. Because adolescents do not feel obligated to tell their parents about personal issues (Smetana, Metzger, Gettman, & Campione-Barr, 2006), they also typically did not use partial disclosure strategies such as omitting important details that parents would want to know (Smetana et al., 2009; Tasopoulos-Chan, Smetana, & Yau, 2009). In our study of Chinese-American, Mexican-American, and European-American youth, information about personal activities was managed primarily by telling their parents (and particularly their fathers) only when asked (Tasopoulos-Chan et al., 2009).

Thus, research on adolescent-parent conflict and adolescents' management of information with parents both suggest that early adolescence and especially middle adolescence might be particular periods of difficulty in adolescent-parent relationships. Conflicts are on the rise, as are attempts to manage and conceal information from parents. It is possible that this simply reflects changes in opportunity. After all, most adolescents in the United States are able to obtain drivers' licenses at these ages, thus increasing their opportunities to roam far from home and engage in risky behavior. And there is clear evidence that risky behaviors, such as experimenting with alcohol and illegal substances, become more normative in middle adolescence. But as discussed later, there also may be other developmental factors at work.

PEER INFLUENCE

Another explanation has to do with the role of peers. Daddis (2008) has proposed that adolescents' friends influence their desires for more autonomy and personal control and that adolescents use friends as a reference to gauge how much autonomy is appropriate. Studying primarily European-American, middle-class, early and middle adolescent close friend dyads,

Daddis (2008) examined adolescents' perceptions of different sources of influence, including the self, friends, parents, other adults, and the media. Consistent with the studies of legitimate parental authority just discussed, adolescents viewed parents as the primary influence on their beliefs about who should control conventional and prudential issues. However, teenagers viewed their friends as influencing their thinking about personal and multifaceted issues. Indeed, when different sources of influence were compared, Daddis (2008) reported that adolescents viewed their friends as having twice as much influence as parents in deciding who should control personal issues. Parental influence over personal issues was greater among middle than high school students, suggesting that parents' influence declines with age. Adolescents relied much less on their own judgments than on their friends, although their reliance on their own judgments increased with age. Friends were seen as influencing thinking about personal authority primarily by setting standards. Adolescents compared the amount of decision-making control they had with what their close friends were allowed to do. Middle adolescents were more likely than early adolescents to use their friends as a metric for deciding what should be personal and up to them to decide. Less often, but more among middle adolescents than early adolescents, teens viewed their friends as offering advice.

In a further study, Daddis (in press) more directly tested the effects of peer influence on adolescents' autonomy seeking. He compared adolescents' perceptions of their own autonomy with their perceptions of how much autonomy their peers had to make decisions regarding different types of issues. As reviewed elsewhere (Smetana, 2011), Daddis asserted that much of the push for greater autonomy occurs over prudential and multifaceted issues; adolescents seek to wrest control of these issues from parents and with age, increasingly view them as personal. (This assertion regarding prudential issues is consistent with the research on adolescents' management of information about their activities, which showed that adolescents often took prudential matters into their own hands. It is also consistent with trends showing that with age, prudential issues are more likely to be conceptualized by teens as personal; Smetana, 2011). Daddis found that adolescents desired more autonomy over multifaceted and prudential issues when they believed that their peers had more autonomy over these issues than they did, but only if their own levels of autonomy were low. When adolescents reported having more autonomy in family decision making regarding these issues, peers' autonomy (relative to their own levels) had no influence. Moreover, adolescents typically overestimated how much autonomy their peers had, particularly over moral, conventional, and prudential issues. Their assessments of their peers' autonomy over multifaceted and personal issues were more real-istic. This provides some support for the notion that adolescents' desires for greater autonomy come partly from their perceptions of how much freedom their peers have. These findings also are consistent with the broader litera-ture on peer relationships, which has shown that conformity to peers and the importance of crowds peak during middle adolescence.

It is worth noting that no matter how much autonomy adolescents want, it is parents who actually decide how much autonomy adolescents should have. In a longitudinal study, Daddis and Smetana (2005) examined the influence of mothers' and middle adolescents' expectations regarding the desired pacing of autonomy over various personal and prudential issues on family decision making about these same issues three years later (Daddis & Smetana, 2005). Only mothers' – but not teens' – autonomy expectations influenced subsequent autonomy. Furthermore, the effects were domain-specific. That is, middle adolescents whose mothers had later expectations for their autonomy over personal issues had less autonomy over these issues (but not prudential issues) three years later, in late adolescence. The same was true for prudential issues. That is, mothers' expectations for the desired pacing of autonomy over prudential issues, as assessed in middle adoles-cence, influenced late adolescents' subsequent autonomy over prudential issues. However, mothers' expectations regarding the desired pacing of autonomy over personal issues – but not prudential issues – influenced how much autonomy over multifaceted issues teens had later on. Therefore, ado-lescents may desire more autonomy and construct broader boundaries of their authority, rely on their friends as metrics of how much autonomy they believe they deserve, and push for more autonomy in situations of conflict, but parents guide the eventual granting of autonomy.

DEVELOPMENTAL CHANGES IN PERSONAL CONCEPTS

Very little research has examined changes with age in children's concep-tions of self and personal issues. There is some evidence indicating that adolescents' self-understanding and concepts of personal choice change over the course of adolescence, but not necessarily in a smooth and linear way. Indeed, it appears that middle adolescence is a period of vulnerabil-ity and challenge in the development of these concepts. Nucci (1996, 2001, 2008) has examined European-American middle-class children's and ado-lescents' understanding of personal concepts. He has shown that the more behavioral notions of personal issues (manifested in terms of exercising choice and maintaining control over personal activities) evident during middle childhood take a more psychological turn during adolescence. Early adolescents become increasingly concerned with the need to maintain privacy, with differentiating the self from others, and with establishing a unique identity. This is expressed in terms of a desire for freedom of choice and the ability to be different from others. Early adolescents express worry about the loss of self and identity by conforming too much to the crowd, while trying to differentiate themselves from peers.

During middle adolescence, however, a new awareness of the "true self" emerges. Middle adolescents attempt to align their inner self with their more public persona. Exercising control over personal issues and making personal decisions become a way to understand and express their true selves. Also, adolescents begin to be sensitive to the aspects of the self that they wish to keep private. Therefore, parental behaviors that are perceived as attempts to violate adolescents' privacy may become particularly troubling during middle adolescence. Conflicts may increase in intensity and information management may be on the rise during middle adolescence because adolescents may feel that there is more at stake in their disputes.

In a similar vein, Harter and Monsour (1992) have documented that multiple selves proliferate during adolescence. These researchers claim that multiple role-related selves first emerge during early adolescence. Teenagers come to see that they act differently and express different characteristics in different situations and in different roles (for instance, with parents versus peers). Early adolescents may view the self in different and even contradictory ways in different relationships, but they are not aware of the inconsistencies in their self-descriptions. Therefore, these contradictions are not troubling.

During middle adolescence, however, adolescents become more aware of contradictions in their self-descriptions. These are subjectively experienced as conflicts and confusions. Harter (2006) has focused more on the intrapsychic dimensions of conflict, but it is possible that confusions in adolescents' attempt to resolve the contradictory aspects also lead to increased conflict with parents. Furthermore, Harter (2006) has made connections between these intrapsychic conflicts of middle adolescence, to which girls are more prone, and girls' increased risks for depression, which also increase at this age.

Both Harter and Monsour (1992) and Nucci (2001, 2008) view late adolescence and emerging adulthood as resolving some of the inconsistencies or dualities of self and personal issues that arise during middle adolescence. Harter and Monsour (1992) claim that during late adolescence and emerging adulthood, youth resolve the contradictory aspects of their self-portraits as they become integrated into a more abstract, higher-order construction.

Likewise, according to Nucci, personal concepts are further transformed during late adolescence. They move from notions of a true self or essence to a view of the self as labile and constantly evolving and changing in the process of making personal choices. Control over personal issues becomes important to coordinating the self-system and constructing an internally consistent whole.

COORDINATIONS ACROSS DOMAINS

The notion that middle adolescence is a time of particular vulnerability compared to earlier and later in adolescence is echoed in several studies examining adolescents' ability to coordinate moral, conventional, and personal concepts. For instance, emerging research suggests that middle adolescence is a time of uncertainty and ambiguity in the development of adolescents' moral thinking. In an ongoing investigation, Nucci and Turiel (2007, 2009) examined children and adolescents' moral reasoning and their ability to weigh different types of concerns in straightforward as well as multifaceted situations. In straightforward moral situations (where there are no competing goals), there was little ambiguity in moral judgments. Across ages, children and adolescents uniformly endorsed the wrongness of harming others and the need to help others.

These researchers also found age-related but nonlinear changes in moral thinking. They found what appeared to be a U-shaped pattern of moral growth. Compared to late childhood and late adolescence, middle adolescence appeared to be a period of particular difficulty and vulnerability characterized by uncertainty in moral thinking. Adolescents (fourteen-year-olds) were better able than younger children to consider new features of moral situations, but their attempts to achieve more complex integrations of moral thought resulted in instability in their thinking. In particular, early to middle adolescents' attempts to establish boundaries of personal jurisdiction resulted in their overapplication of the personal domain in morally ambiguous contexts. This was not evident in evaluations of prototypical moral issues, in more neutral situations, or situations where transgressions were depicted as provoked. It was only apparent when adolescents attempted to coordinate reasoning about harm and helping in hypothetical situations depicting vulnerable individuals. In attempting to coordinate moral notions of rights with their developing notions of the personal domain, adolescents overextended the personal aspects of these ambiguous situations and ignored their moral dimensions. Thus, in these circumstances, they gave more weight to personal prerogatives and personal goals in middle adolescence relative to pre- or late adolescence. As a fourteen-year-old in Nucci and Turiel's study stated,

"I think she has a right to do what she wants to [about stealing]. Because it is once again his decision to do what he wants." By late adolescence, youth were once again able to distinguish personal choices from conceptions of rights. They also became better able to coordinate the boundaries of the personal and moral domains.

Similar findings have been obtained in a recent large longitudinal survey study of adolescents' perceptions of an individual's right to engage in risky behaviors that are potentially harmful to health (Flanagan, Stout, & Gallay, 2008). These researchers asked fifth- through twelfth-graders to evaluate a set of beliefs pertaining to what they referred to as individual rights, but which were consistent with what I have referred to here as the personal domain. The beliefs pertained to doing what one wants with his or her body, smoking or drinking as a personal choice, and having a right to smoke because it is seen as only harming oneself. These researchers also assessed what they referred to as public health beliefs (for instance, that the government should make laws to protect society against drunk driving or that if something is bad for health, the government should tell individuals to avoid it). Inasmuch as these issues pertain to others' welfare, they can be seen as moral issues, but they also include social-conventional concerns with the regulatory aspects of government. Individual rights and public health beliefs were found to change with age, but in different ways.

Endorsement of individual rights (personal choices) was relatively low across ages, but both cross-sectional and longitudinal analyses suggested that beliefs about the right to control the personal domain increased with age across adolescence. However, there appeared to be a curvilinear relationship with age in adolescents' endorsement of society's ability to control adolescents' risky behaviors (that is, public health beliefs). Again, both cross-sectional and longitudinal analyses converged to demonstrate a decline in middle adolescence, as compared to early or late adolescence, in endorsement of those beliefs.

The researchers concluded that by late adolescence, youth develop a more sophisticated conception of health beliefs. In their view, this involved a coordination between individual rights (individuals' personal choice to experiment with substances) and "a recognition of the need for laws enacted by government that constrain individuals' rights in the interest of a larger public good" (Flanagan et al., 2008, p. 831). As Nucci and Turiel (2007, 2009) found, middle adolescence involves an overextension of the personal domain and what Flanagan et al., (2008) referred to as "an ardent commitment to personal rights as a basis for making decisions" (p. 831). It was not until late adolescence that youth were able to coordinate these two sets of beliefs.

CONCLUSIONS

These findings and their implications for adolescent-parent relationships will need to be explored in further research. But it is interesting to note that difficulties in resolving the inconsistencies of multiple selves, of integrating notions of a true self with exercising personal choices, and of coordinating the boundaries of the personal and moral domains all coincide with increases in the intensity of conflicts with parents and with managing and concealing information from parents. There is general agreement that conflict and information management are temporary perturbations that reflect the outward reach of autonomy. Earlier, I claimed that adolescent-parent conflict represents parents' and adolescents' failure to coordinate their perspectives on issues. However, the studies just reviewed further suggest that adolescent-parent conflict also may arise from adolescents' inability to coordinate personal, moral, and social-conventional concepts. Both adolescent-parent relationships and the development of social reasoning are complex and fraught with both challenges and opportunities. Relationships with parents clearly improve once adolescents leave home. But resolutions to problems in their relationships also may be achieved as late adolescents develop the ability to integrate and coordinate different social concepts. By the end of adolescence, youth appear to develop more nuanced, contextually sensitive, and integrated social, moral, and personal understandings of their social world.

REFERENCES

Adams, R., & Laursen, B. (2001). The organization and dynamics of adolescent conflict with parents and friends. *Journal of Marriage & the Family, 63*, 97–110.

Collins, W. A., & Laursen, B. (1992). Conflict and relationships during adolescence. In C. U. Shantz & W. W. Hartup (Eds.), *Conflict in child and adolescent development* (pp. 216–241). Cambridge: Cambridge University Press.

(2004). Parent-adolescent relationships and influences. In R. M. Lerner & L. Steinberg (Ed.), *Handbook of adolescent psychology* (2nd Ed., pp. 331–361). Hoboken, NJ: Wiley.

Cumsille, P., Darling, N., Flaherty, B. P., & Martinez, M. L. (2006). Chilean adolescents' beliefs about the legitimacy of parental authority: Individual and age-related difference. *International Journal of Behavioral Development, 30*, 97–106.

(2009). Heterogeneity and change in the patterning of adolescents' perceptions of the legitimacy of parental authority: A latent transition model. *Child Development, 80*, 418–432.

Daddis, C. (2008). Influence of close friends on the boundaries of adolescent personal authority. *Journal of Research on Adolescence, 18*, 75–98.

(in press). Desire for increased autonomy and adolescents' perceptions of peer autonomy: "Everyone else can; Why can't I?" *Child Development.*

Daddis, C., & Smetana, J. G. (2005). Middle class African American families' expectations for adolescents' behavioral autonomy. *International Journal of Behavioral Development, 29,* 371–381.

Darling, N., Cumsille, P., & Martinez, M. L. (2008). Individual differences in adolescents' beliefs about the legitimacy of parental authority and their own obligation to obey: A longitudinal investigation. *Child Development, 79,* 1103–1118.

Finkenauer, C., Engels, R. C. M. E., & Meeus, W. (2002). Keeping secrets from parents: Advantages and disadvantages of secrecy in adolescence. *Journal of Youth and Adolescence, 2,* 123–136.

Flanagan, C. A., Stout, M., & Gallay, L. S. (2008). It's my body and none of your business: Developmental changes in adolescents' perceptions of rights concerning health. *Journal of Social Issues, 64,* 815–834.

Fuligni, A. J. (1998). Authority, autonomy, and parent-adolescent conflict and cohesion: A study of adolescents from Mexican, Chinese, Filipino, and European backgrounds. *Developmental Psychology, 34,* 782–792.

Furman, W., & Buhrmester, D. (1985). Children's perceptions of the personal relationships in their social networks. *Developmental Psychology, 21,* 1016–1024.

(1992). Age and sex in perceptions of networks of personal relationships. *Child Development, 63,* 103–115.

Harter, S. (2006). The self. In N. Eisenberg (Ed.), *Handbook of child psychology, 6th Ed., Vol. 3: Social, emotional, and personality development* (William Damon, Series Editor; pp. 505–570). New York: Wiley.

Harter, S., & Monsour, A. (1992). Developmental analysis of conflict caused by opposing attributes in the adolescent self-portrait. *Developmental Psychology, 28,* 251–260.

Holmbeck, G. N. (1996). A model of family relational transformations during the transition to adolescence: Parent-adolescent conflict and adaptation. In J. A. Graber, J. Brooks-Gunn, & A. C. Petersen (Eds.), *Transitions through adolescence: Interpersonal domains and context* (pp. 167–199). Mahwah, NJ: Erlbaum.

Keijsers, L., Branje, S. J., Frijns, T., Finkenauer, C., & Meeus, W. (2010). Gender differences in keeping secrets from parents in adolescence. *Developmental Psychology, 46,* 293–298.

Keijsers, L., Frijns, T., Branje, S. J., & Meeus, W. (2009). Developmental links of adolescent disclosure, parental solicitation, and control with delinquency: Moderation with parental support. *Developmental Psychology, 45,* 1314–1327.

Laird, R. D., & Marrero, M. D. (2010). Information management and behavior problems: Is concealing misbehavior necessarily a sign of trouble? *Journal of Adolescence, 33,* 297–308.

Larson, R. W., Moneta, G., Richards, M. H., & Wilson, S. (2002). Continuity, stability, and change in daily emotional experience across adolescence. *Child Development, 73,* 1151–1165.

Larson, R. W., & Richards, M. H. (1994). *Divergent realities: The emotional lives of mothers, fathers, and adolescents.* New York: Basic Books.

Laursen, B., & Collins, W. A. (1994). Interpersonal conflict during adolescence. *Psychological Bulletin, 115*, 197–209.

(2009). Parent-child relationships during adolescence. In R. L. Lerner & L. Steinberg (Eds.), *Handbook of adolescent psychology* (3rd Ed., Vol. 2, pp. 3–42). New York: John Wiley & Sons.

Laursen, B., Coy, K., & Collins, W. A. (1998). Reconsidering changes in parent-child conflict across adolescence: A meta-analysis. *Child Development, 69*, 817–832.

Nucci, L. P. (1996). Morality and personal freedom. In E. S. Reed, E. Turiel, & T. Brown (Eds.), *Values and knowledge* (pp. 41–60). Mahwah, NJ: Erlbaum.

(2001). *Education in the moral domain.* Cambridge: Cambridge University Press.

(2008). *Nice is not enough: Facilitating moral development.* New York: Pearson.

Nucci, L. P., & Smetana, J. G. (1996). Mothers' concepts of young children's areas of personal freedom. *Child Development, 67*, 1870–1886.

Nucci, L. P., & Turiel. E. (2007). *Development in the moral domain: The role of conflict and relationships in children's and adolescents' welfare and harm judgments.* Paper presented at the Biennial Meetings of the Society for Research in Child Development, Boston, MA.

(2009). Capturing the complexity of moral development and education. *Mind, Brain, and Education, 3*, 151–159.

Nucci, L. P., & Weber, E. K. (1995). Social interactions in the home and the development of young children's conceptions of the personal. *Child Development, 66*, 1438–1452.

Smetana, J. G. (1989). Adolescents' and parents' reasoning about actual family conflict. *Child Development, 60*, 1052–1067.

(1995). Morality in context: Abstractions, ambiguities, and applications. In R. Vasta (Ed.), *Annals of child development* (Vol. 10, pp. 83–130). London: Jessica Kingsley Publishers.

(1996). Adolescent-parent conflict: Implications for adaptive and maladaptive development. In D. Cicchetti & S. L. Toth (Eds.), *Rochester symposium on developmental psychopathology, Vol. VII: Adolescence: Opportunities and challenges* (pp. 1–46). Rochester, NY: University of Rochester Press.

(2002). Culture, autonomy, and personal jurisdiction in adolescent-parent relationships. In H. W. Reese & R. Kail (Eds.), *Advances in child development and behavior* (Vol. 29, pp. 51–87). New York: Academic Press.

(2006). Social domain theory: Consistencies and variations in children's moral and social judgments. In M. Killen & J. G. Smetana (Eds.), *Handbook of Moral Development* (pp. 119–154). Mahwah, NJ: Erlbaum.

(2011). *Adolescents, families, and social development: How teens construct their worlds.* West Sussex: Wiley-Blackwell.

Smetana, J. G., Campione-Barr, N., & Daddis, C. (2004). Developmental and longitudinal antecedents of family decision-making: Defining health behavioral autonomy for African American adolescents. *Child Development, 75*, 1418–1434.

Smetana, J. G., Campione-Barr, N., & Metzger, A. (2006). Adolescent development in interpersonal and societal contexts. *Annual Review of Psychology, 57*, 255–284.

Smetana, J. G., Daddis, C., & Chuang, S. S. (2003). "Clean your room!" : A longitudinal investigation of adolescent-parent conflict in middle class African American families. *Journal of Adolescent Research, 18*, 631–650.

Smetana, J. G., Metzger, A., Gettman, D. C., & Campione-Barr, N. (2006). Disclosure and secrecy in adolescent-parent relationships. *Child Development, 77*, 201–217.

Smetana, J. G., Villalobos, M., Rogge, R. D., & Tasopoulos-Chan, M. (2010). Keeping secrets from parents: Daily variations among poor, urban adolescents. *Journal of Adolescence, 33*, 321–331.

Smetana, J. G., Villalobos, M., Tasopoulos-Chan, M., Gettman, D. C., & Campione-Barr, N. (2009). Early and middle adolescents' disclosure to parents about activities in different domains. *Journal of Adolescence, 32*, 693–713.

Tasopoulos-Chan, M., Smetana, J. G., & Yau, J. Y. (2009). How much do I tell thee? Strategic management of information with parents among American adolescents from Mexican, Chinese, and European backgrounds. *Journal of Family Psychology, 23*, 364–374.

Turiel, E. (1983). *The development of social knowledge: Morality and convention.* Cambridge: Cambridge University Press.

(2002). *The culture of morality: Social development, context, and conflict.* Cambridge: Cambridge University Press.

(2006). The development of morality. In N. Eisenberg (Ed.), *Handbook of child psychology, 6th Ed., Vol. 3: Social, emotional, and personality development* (William Damon, Series Editor; pp. 789–857). New York: Wiley.

Yau, J., & Smetana, J. G. (1996). Adolescent-parent conflict among Chinese adolescents in Hong Kong. *Child Development, 67*, 1262–1275.

(2003). Adolescent-parent conflict in Hong Kong and Shenzhen: A comparison of youth in two cultural contexts. *International Journal of Behavioral Development, 27*, 201–211.

Yau, J. Y., Tasopoulos-Chan, M., & Smetana, J. G. (2009). Disclosure to parents about everyday activities among American adolescents from Mexican, Chinese, and European backgrounds. *Child Development, 80*, 1481–1498.

Zhang, W., & Fuligni, A. J. (2006). Authority, autonomy, and family relationships among adolescents in urban and rural China. *Journal of Research on Adolescence, 16*, 527–537.

8

Representations, Process, and Development: A New Look at Friendship in Early Adolescence

WILLIAM M. BUKOWSKI, MELISSA SIMARD,
AND MARIE EVE DUBOIS

Concordia University (Montréal, Québec)

LUZ STELLA LOPEZ

Universidad Del Norte (Barranquilla, Colombia)

For many early adolescents, friendship functions as a centerpiece of daily experience. Early adolescents spend time and interact with their friends in environments that are real, electronic, or virtual. Together they share a range of experiences including achievement-related and social events at school, the affective ups and downs associated with family life, and the multifaceted experiences associated with adjusting to new freedoms and new internal states and desires. The importance of friendship during this period has not been lost on writers and filmmakers. The best known works of fiction about early adolescents typically tell a story about how a person of this age makes his or her way through life in the company of his or her friends. The Harry Potter stories are the best examples of this genre of literature. Millions and millions of readers have been captivated by the stories of the experiences that Harry shares with his friends – Ron and Hermoine – at their school. These stories, and many others, are exemplary in their depictions of the challenges and opportunities associated with friendship for early adolescent boys and girls.

The challenges and opportunities posed by friendship in early adolescence have been well recognized by developmental psychologists. Research on friendship has been a mainstay of research on social development for more than a century (Bukowski & Sippola, 2005). This research has been motivated by multiple interests. Three research goals have been especially prominent: (a) to identify what friendship consists of, (b) to assess how friendship affects development and well-being, and (c) to examine the intersection between friendship and risk status. Attention has been devoted to each of these goals.

Insofar as one needs to know what one is studying before it can be measured in a way that would reveal its developmental significance, attempts to identify the features of friendship have typically preceded efforts to identify the effects of friendship and its association with risk. Accordingly these three research streams have not run completely in parallel. Instead, research on the features of friendship has preceded research on the general effects of friendship, which, in turn has informed research on friendship and risk.

Research on friendship in early adolescence has been typically based on a multifaceted idea. The three components that make up this idea follow directly from the three goals that have motivated research on friendship. This idea is that (a) because friendship relations offer specific provisions that can not be obtained in other forms of relationship experience (Furman & Robins, 1985; Hartup, 1979), (b) they provide unique forms of experience that have immediate effects on well-being (Berndt, 1982; Demir & Urberg, 2004; Mannarino, 1978; Newcomb & Bagwell, 1996), and (c) that these effects will be stronger for early adolescents than for other boys and girls who are "at risk" for negative outcomes (e.g., early adolescent from nonoptimal family contexts). Together these three facets point to the opportunities and challenges of friendship. The opportunities offered by friendship are the unique experiences it provides. It has been argued that friendship in early adolescence differs in fundamental ways from the friendships experienced at younger ages and from relationship experiences with parents. Compared with the friendships of younger children, friendships in early adolescence are more likely to provide opportunities for closeness and intimacy and less likely to be play-based; compared with relationships with parents, they are more likely to be characterized by equality and balance. In regard to the challenges of friendship, if it is the case that friendship experiences are necessary for well-being, then developing positive friendship relations that are characterized by closeness and equality is a critical challenge for early adolescents. According to the risk component of the previously stated idea, having friends is expected to be of greater importance for early adolescents whose individual characteristics (e.g., being prone to anxiety) or social experiences (e.g., being victimized) put them at an increased probability for negative outcomes (e.g., depressed affect).

Friendship also poses opportunities and challenges for researchers who study it. The opportunity it provides is clear. It offers a rich domain for studying the intersection between the personal and the social. The challenge is also clear. Persons who study friendship need to identify its central features and to develop ways of measuring them so that one can assess individual differences in friendship experience. Then, of course, one needs to design studies to assess how friendship experience is related to well-being. The progress on each of these challenges has been well catalogued already (Bukowski, Motzoi, & Meyer, 2008). Researchers have been successful at developing measures of the features that characterize friendship (Furman & Buhrmester, 1985) and at demonstrating the effects that friendship has on adjustment (Bukowski, Brendgen, & Vitaro, 2006). The lion's share of these studies have typically employed a single index of friendship that has been used as a predictor of subsequent measures of well-being. Research has shown also that the effects of friendship can be especially strong for at-risk early adolescents (Hodges, Mallone, & Perry, 1997). Together these studies have produced impressive evidence that friendship matters.

In spite of the apparent richness of existing research on friendship, it is important to step back and ask whether current research on friendship during early adolescence has truly captured the dynamics of friendship and well-being during this period. When we look at current research on friendship and try to think about it from a specifically developmental perspective, we wonder if the practices that have been used to study friendship, especially the use of single indicators to measure individual differences, have adequately represented the richness of friendships. From this perspective it appears that many basic questions about friendship in early adolescence remain unanswered. These questions are related to each of the three facets that make up the powerful idea that has motivated research on friendship. Our particular concern is that there has been a lack of interest in seeing friendship from a process orientation in which some aspects of friendship lead to others. We not only see these dynamic processes as the central challenge of friendship, but we regard a process-oriented approach as important way for understanding how friendship intersects with risk status. This chapter is an effort to explain a process-oriented approach to friendship.

The chapter is organized in the following way. First we address the question of which features are most central to friendship. This discussion derives from several perspectives. Next we discuss ideas about the origins and emergence of friendship. The point of this discussion is that friendship is a dynamic process in which some features are a consequence of others. The central point of this discussion is that one needs to take a process-oriented perspective. Finally we turn our attention to the concept of risk. Our particular interest is to assess differences in the processes of friendship for two groups of early adolescents who are known to be at risk for maladjustment. These at-risk early adolescents are those who are from families of either upper or lower socioeconomic status. The first section of the chapter offers a basic review of research on representations of friendship.

FEATURES OF FRIENDSHIP IN EARLY ADOLESCENCE: EVOLVING REPRESENTATIONS OF FRIENDSHIP

Efforts to identify the key features of friendship have been a long-standing activity of friendship researchers. Although this area is not as active now as it was twenty-five or thirty-five years ago, the findings continue to inform current research on friendship. This older literature consisted mostly of qualitative studies whose purpose was to understand how representations of friendship changed with age. It is important to recognize from the outset that the goal of these studies was to identify the characteristics that children and early adolescents ascribe to friendship. Typically the questions used in these qualitative studies referred specifically to the features that children believe comprise friendship. They did not ask where these features came from or how they were related to each other. We see this emphasis on the multiple features that define friendship to be a strength of this literature and the lack of attention to process as a weakness.

The ideas underlying friendship research derive from several theories. These theories include the ideas of social psychiatrists such as Sullivan (1953), sociologists such as Mead (1934), attachment theorists such as Blatz (1966), and social psychologists such as Weiss (1974). There is also a very rich set of ideas in the ancient (e.g., Aristotle, 1973) and not-so-ancient (Blum, 1980; Friedman, 1989; Raymond, 1986) philosophical literature about friendship (Bukowski & Sippola, 1996). Both old and new ideas from philosophy imply that friendship has both self-involved and other-involved features. These self-involved features concern the pleasure and value that result from having a friend, whereas the other-involved features refer to one's dedication and loyalty to one's friend. Aristotle and his recent followers believed that the more self-involved features of friendship were related to pleasure. Beneficial interactions were the transitory and superficial features of friendship, whereas the other-focused concepts of friendship that emphasized the relationship per se were those that had had the larger and more enduring significance.

Although the ideas of philosophers and of other theorists can stimulate our own thinking abut friendship, their value for research on friendship is limited if these same concepts are not used by children and adolescents when they think about their friends. Accordingly, an important theme of friendship research was to assess children's friendship conceptions. Much of this original work was inspired by the Piagetian concepts of representation and construction (Selman 1981). Its goals were to assess how children constructed the concept of friendship and how these constructions changed with age. The findings showed clearly that representations of friendship change during childhood and early adolescence. In these studies, researchers have used questions such as "What is a best friend?" (Youniss, 1980), or "What do you expect from a best friend?" (Bigelow, 1977). One frequent response to the questions was not dependent on age. Children of all ages have claimed that high levels of shared activities, affection, and reciprocal "giving-and-taking" are basic features of friendship (Hartup & Stevens, 1997). Research has shown that young children's conceptions of a friend are typically based in the here-and-now and are not easily separated from social interaction. By the early school-age years, children conceive of friendship as more than just shared play. For these children, friendship transcends specific activity and is enduring over time. Nevertheless, at this age, friendship continues to be based on instrumental and concrete considerations of pleasure and utility. Bigelow (1977), for example, has shown that at the start of middle childhood (age seven to eight years), children's concept of friendship often involves the notions of rewards and costs – friends are individuals who are rewarding to be with, and nonfriends are peers who are difficult or uninteresting to interact with. This conception of friendship evolves across middle childhood and early adolescence. By age ten or eleven years, most children recognize the importance of shared values and shared social understanding for friendship. Friends at this age are expected to stick up for and be loyal to one another.

By age eleven or twelve years, children's concept of a friend includes the view that friends share similar interests, are required to make active attempts to understand each other, and are willing to engage in self-disclosure. The importance of interpersonal support becomes stronger as well. With age, children recognize the higher level of supportiveness between friends and nonfriends (Berndt & Perry, 1986). Moreover, children's descriptions of their friendships indicate that loyalty, self-disclosure, and trust are more frequently included in representations of friendship as children enter early adolescence (Berndt, 2004, 2002), especially among girls (Berndt, 1986; Berndt & Perry, 1986; Buhrmester, 1990; Strough, Swenson, Cheng, 2001). At this age, both boys and girls begin to possess more intimate knowledge of their friends (Berndt, 2002). They begin to describe their friends in a more differentiated and integrated manner (Peevers & Secord, 1973) and see them as more exclusive and individualized (Smollar & Youniss, 1982). It is important to recognize that as children develop, they do not cast away their representations of friendship as consisting of shared play, common activities, and mutual affection, but they increasingly recognize the importance of intimacy and loyalty (Berndt, 1996). A study of school-age children's drawings of their friends show that at this age friends are perceived as sharing many basic activity interests while at the same time being able to show their loyalty and closeness to each other (Pinto, Bombi, & Cordoli, 1997).

Summary

At least three important points can be gleaned from theses findings. The first is that children's and adolescents' representations of friendship are multidimensional. They include a set of interrelated features rather than a single critical factor. Second, these representations evolve. During early childhood, they are concrete and self-focused; by early adolescence, they are increasingly abstract and relational. It is important to recognize that two types of change are seen in these age differences. One type of change concerns a process of accumulation. With age, new features are incorporated into the concept of what defines a friendship. Features such as shared liking and common activities that are central to friendship in childhood maintain their place in the friendship representations even as new representations are added. The other type of change concerns a movement away from a self-focused view toward one that is placed in the relationship per se. This change is consistent with the general Piagetian claim that development consists of a movement away from a self-centered perspective. A third central point that can be seen in these findings is that early adolescents are aware of the multidimensional nature of their friendship experiences. By including several features in their descriptions of what constitutes a friendship and by recognizing that some are more significant than others, early adolescents show that they realize that friendship involves different processes and outcomes (e.g, a sense of security or well-being).

BUT WHAT IS THE STUFF OF FRIENDSHIP AND WHAT DOES "IT" MEAN FOR MEASUREMENT?

Children's and adolescents' comments about friendship provide an important source of information about what friendship is. By themselves, however, these comments can provide only so much guidance to investigators who wish to study what it means to have a friend in the school-age and early adolescent periods. The direct use of children's representations to assess friendship poses two challenges. The first is that several features are included in descriptions of friendship, and one needs to decide which of them should be included in a measurement of friendship experience. One cannot measure all aspects. Instead, one has to identify a set of basic concepts that will capture most of the richness in children's and adolescents' comments about what friendship is. Second, one needs to look beyond the comments that children and adolescents make to assess whether the features they refer to are consistent with other reports of what friendship is.

These challenges can be addressed together by looking for parallels between the findings from the friendship conception literature and from two other literatures. One of these consists of observational studies of friendship during childhood and adolescence. The other is the literature on the role of relationships in development. In spite of the different goals and methods of these studies, they share a common purpose of trying to understand what friendship is and how it works to affect development. In our assessment of the research on friendship, we have looked for commonalities among them so as to come up with a set of essential aspects of friendship that one would need to include in a measure of friendship. We have identified five dimensions that, in our view, are critical features of friendship. They are companionship, conflict, help, security, and closeness. Each of the latter three is further divided into two smaller dimensions.

Companionship

In both the conceptual and empirical literatures regarding childhood and adolescent friendships, there has been an emphasis on play, association and companionship. Friendships involve people who do things together. The word "companionship" comes from the Latin word "with bread." This meaning tells us that literally and metaphoriocally friends are people who share the "staff of life." Observational studies of friendship have typically used play or another form of interaction as the observational context (e.g., Newcomb & Brady, 1982). In the conceptual literature on friendship, researchers (Buhrmester & Furman, 1987; Davies 1982; Hinde, 1979; Sullivan, 1953; Furman & Robins, 1985; Selman, 1981; Weiss, 1974) have all, in one way or another, identified play and companionship as a basic feature or component of children's friendship relations. These individuals have argued that opportunities for interaction with a liked peer are a fundamental aspect or basis of what it means to be someone's friend during childhood or early adolescence.

Conflict

In spite of the idyllic views of friendship that can be found in endless number of sappy greeting cards and bad poems, observational studies have shown that friends have more conflicts with each other than they do with other peers (Rubin, Bukowski, & Parker, 2006). Several observational studies have shown that conflict is a frequent salient feature of children's friendships (Adler & Furman, 1988; Hartup, Laursen, Stewart, & Eastenson, 1988; Shantz & Shantz, 1985; Shantz, 1986), and studies of friendship have shown that among children, conflict is a correlate of the continuity of the friendship relation (Berndt, 1982; Gottman, 1983). Conflicts are a likely, if not inevitable, consequence of any relationship that requires decision making. Measures of conflict typically assess the extent to which children can get into fights and arguments with their friends and annoy each other, and that there are disagreements in the friendship relation.

Help

There is a very large literature regarding the role of aid and support in relations (see Belle, 1989; Berndt, 1982; Buhrmester & Furman, 1987; Selman, 1981). Several researchers (Furman & Robbins, 1985; Weiss, 1974) have argued that provisions of aid are an important part of the friendship process. Essentially, friends help each other. Aside from the encouragement for exploration, which is an important part of companionship, friends provide instrumental aid in a variety of domains. The importance of help and aid for friendship is apparent also in children's and early adolescents' evaluations of friendship features (Berndt, 1982; Bigelow, 1977; Bukowski et al., 1987). In the *Friendship Qualities Scale* (Bukowski, Hoza, & Boivin, 1994), help is represented as consisting of two different components. One is called *Aid*, and it is made up of items indicating that mutual help and assistance are features of the friendship relation. The other subscale is called *Protection from Victimization*. The items in this subscale refer to the friend's willingness to come to the child's aid if another child was bothering him or her. Given the fact that nearly all children are at one time or another victimized by peers, this scale is likely to have a great deal of salience for children and early adolescents. Indeed, two independent theoretical accounts of friendship have proposed that a basic function of friendship is to provide protection to children who are at risk for victimization (Davies, 1982; Rizzo, 1989).[1]

Security

Security has been regarded as one of the most central features of friendship. Beginning with the seminal work of Blatz (summarized in Blatz, 1966)

---

[1] Analyses of the psychometric properties of these scales have shown them to have adequate levels of internal consistency and to be largely independent of each other. Similar conditions have been observed with other subscales in the *Friendship Qualities Scale*.

and Salter (Ainsworth) (1940), subsequent perspectives of Coleman (1974), Davies (1982), Douvan and Adelson (1966), and Eichhorn (1980), there has been a great deal of consensus that security is a critical property of children's and adolescents' relationships with their friends. All of these writers have argued that for children and adolescents, two central features of friendship are the impression that their friendships are secure and capable of continuing in spite of problems or conflicts, and the belief that they can trust and rely on their friends. According to these perspectives, friendship has an essentially transcendent quality. It is not based in the here-and-now but instead has an enduring nature that assures its continuity across time and circumstance. Just as a critical feature of formal operations is adolescents' ability to project themselves into the future, a critical feature of adolescent friendship is the extent to which relationships can be seen as experiences that are part of the future as well as the present.

Security has been assessed according to at least two dimensions. In the *Friendship Qualities Scale*, security is indexed with one set of items that refer the existence of a *Reliable Alliance* between friends and another set that refer to the capacity of the friendship to *Transcend Problems*. The primary focus of the items in the reliable alliance subscale is the belief that at times of need, their friend can be relied on and trusted. The items in the transcending problems subscale refer to the belief that if there were a quarrel or a fight or some other form of negative event, the friendship would be strong enough to withstand this problem.

Closeness

It has been pointed out already (e.g., Fine, 1981; Rutter, 1989) that the most persistent themes in the theoretical literature regarding children's and early adolescents' friendship relationships is that these relations are affordances for feelings of acceptance, validation, and attachment. Aside from the typical references to the ideas of Sullivan (1953), Fine (1981) highlighted the work of the "symbolic interactionists" to support an emphasis on closeness. These theorists (Blumer, 1969; Cooley, 1909, 1964; Mead, 1934) have argued that one of the main provisions of relationships is information about the goodness or value of the self. Inherent in their ideas is the notion that the closeness of the affective bond in a friendship relationship gives children and early adolescents the opportunities for reflected appraisal and affection that indicate that they are important to and valued by their friend. This point parallels the central process emphasized by Sullivan (1953) in his well-known theory of childhood and early adolescent friendship relations. The items that comprise the closeness domain in the *Friendship Qualities Scale* refer to the sense of affection or "specialness" that they experience with their friend and the strength of their attachment or bond to their friend. Two distinct sets of items are used. One set of items, called *Affective Bond*, that make up this scale refer to children's feelings about their friend; the other set, called *Reflected Appraisal*, refers to the feelings children derive from the friendship and their impression of how important they are to their friend.

Summary

Identifying the "stuff" of friendship is important for at least two reasons. First, this inquiry helps us understand a fundamentally human relationship. Friendship is a context for human development. It is a relational domain where children and adolescents spend a large proportion of their time regardless of whether they are in the presences of their friends or not. Second, knowing the dimensions that make up friendship for children and adolescents is essential for measurement. Research on friendship requires measures than can capture the factors that are at the heart of this relationship. Effort to develop these measures have consisted of deriving a basic set of friendship characteristics from research on children's descriptions of friendship, observational studies of friendship, as well as theory and research on the developmental significance of friendship. Several features of friendship distilled from this literature have been used as the dimensional characteristics of friendship in well-known measures of friendship. These include assessments of companionship, conflict, help (instrumental aid and protection from victimization), security (transcending problems and trust), and closeness (reliable alliance and affective bond) in the *Friendship Qualities Scale* (Bukowski, Hoza, & Boivin, 1994), as well as assessments of affection, admiration, intimacy, and are included in the *Network of Relationships Inventory* (Furman & Buhrmester, 1985).

We have said already that the assessment of the central features of friendship is a critical step for understanding and accurately measuring friendship. Nevertheless, it is just the first step. The second step consists of understanding how these features are interrelated. The emphasis of this analysis is on structure and organization. Understanding how the features of friendship are structured is important for two reasons. First, it provides further insight into what friendship is and how it functions to affect well-being. Knowing the structure or organization among the features of friendship, one can begin to understand the process of friendship. Second, an emphasis on structure in conjunction with representations provides a different way of thinking about individual differences in friendship, especially as these differences may be related contextual variations and risk factors. Specifically, a structural approach that is focused on associations between variables provides dynamic means of understanding differences between adolescents from different circumstances. Issues related to a structural approach are discussed in the next section.

A STRUCTURAL OR PROCESS APPROACH TO THE FEATURES OF FRIENDSHIP

In nearly every domain of psychology, researchers face the choice between using measures that are narrow and specific or the ones that are broad and general. The option one chooses depends on multiple methodological and theoretical considerations. The presence of many methodological challenges and inconveniences in the absence of strong theoretical considerations has typically led researchers who study friendship to use broad indices of friendship rather than more specific indices. For example, in our own work (Gauze, Bukowski, Aquan-Assee, & Sippola, 1996), we have tended to use a single measure of friendship quality that was an aggregate of more specific measures (e.g., companionship, help, security, and closeness). Others who use the Network of Relationships Inventory (NRI) have also tended to follow Furman and Buhrmester's (1985) recommendations to combine the positive aspects of friendship together to create a single omnibus measure. These decisions have positive and negative consequences. By combining scores on specific measures to form a single index, one loses the opportunity to assess which aspects of friendship matter the most. Perhaps more importantly, it overlooks the distinctions that children and adolescents make between different features of friendship. In other words, the use of aggregated scores does not capture the specific forms of richness that children see in their friendships. Nevertheless, this practice presents some advantages. Dealing with just one measure instead of several presents fewer opportunities for the statistical and interpretive problems that can arise when one includes multiple, highly intercorrelated measures in the same model. Wariness of this problem was especially warranted at a time when multivariate methods were not as well developed as they are currently.

Another reason to use broadband scores was the insensitivity to the availability of a model that would guide thinking about how to structure the associations between different aspects of friendship. When measures of friendship were initially developed and put into practice, ideas about how they could be organized to fit a conceptually meaningful model were not as well known as they are today. Currently, the study of peer relationships has been organized according to a multilevel model that includes three interrelated levels of social complexity, specifically the individual, the dyad, and the group (Rubin et al., 1998, 2006). Friendship is the best-known peer experience at the level of the dyad. According to Hinde's (1987) initial conceptualization of this three-level model, dyadic experiences can be divided into *interactions* and *relationships*. *Interaction* refers to the social exchanges that occur between two individuals. They include the forms of action that the two partners engage in together. Interactions do not need to be equal or balanced. For example, help is a kind of interaction in the sense that it a type of action that occurs between two persons even though one person may do more helping than the other. *Relationships* refer to the meanings, expectations, and emotions that derive from a succession of interactions between two individuals known to each other. Although they both refer to the dyad, interactions are overt and observable; relationships are internal.

An important part of Hinde's model is that interactions (i.e., action) are antecedent to relationships (i.e., internal representations). This explicit organization has two important implications for the study of friendship. The first is that one should be cautious about mixing measures of interactions and relationships. Insofar as they are different aspects of dyadic experience, their combination would lead to a conceptually heterogeneous measure whose meaning is not specific. A second implication is more important. By identifying interactions as antecedent to relationships, it implies a path model in which interactions are predictors of relationships. This organization or structure indicates that the various aspects of friendship are not just related to each other but that some (i.e., interactions) precede others (i.e., relationships). The meaning of this depiction for friendship research is that instead of forcing the features of friendship together to create a single broadband score, one should organize them according to this path model.

Three aspects of this structural organization deserve our attention. The first is that it is a case in which ontogeny is recapitulated in a dyadic experience. That is, the same changes that are seen in children's and early adolescents' representations of friendship (i.e., the ontogeny of friendship) are seen also in the development of particular friendship relationships. We have shown earlier that the developmental path of conceptions of friendship indicates that at earlier ages, there is an emphasis on interactions, which evolves toward an emphasis on internalized representations based on relationships. This same pathway is an explicit feature of Hinde's model of the development of experiences at the level of the dyad. Specifically, interactions come first and relationships follow. This same progression – that is, action followed by internal representations – is at the heart of the Piagetian model of development.

The second part of this proposed organization that deserves our attention concerns the presumed differences in the significance of interactions and relationships. According to Hinde, relationship features of friendship have more significance and meaning than the interaction-based features. If this is the case, and if the meaning-laden aspects of friendship are those that contribute to adolescents' sense of well-being, then one can expect that the association between measures of interaction and measure of well-being will be mediated by the relationship measures.

A third aspect of this model is that it raises an important potential source of difference between individuals. The typical approach to the study of the effect of friendship on well-being has focused on the association between indices of friendship quality and measures of adjustment. This approach is essentially quantitative. It is based on the premise that high scores on measures of friendship quality will be associated with high scores on measures of well-being. It also assumes that there will be an orderly and progressive flow from measures of interactions to measures of relationships to measures of well-being. It is important to recognize that the associations in the model may be as meaningful as the levels of friendship quality. Having positive interactions may not matter unless they lead to positive relationships; having positive relationships is presumed to be important because these experiences will lead to well-being. Accordingly, the study of friendship needs to go beyond a consideration of amounts by examining whether the presumed links between interactions, relationships, and well-being are the same for all persons. Indeed, in addition to limited amounts of interaction and of relationship features in friendship, a further source of risk or variations in friendship effects may be a lack of association from interaction to relationships and from relationship experiences to well-being. That is, risk may derive from an inability to translate interactions into relationships and to derive well-being from having positive relationships experiences.

Summary

The study of friendship needs to consider representations and structures, especially as they are associated with development. Typically friendship research has relied more on the former than the latter, and it has done so via a reliance on broadband measures. Aside from the limitations that derive from the lack of conceptual specificity in broad-based measures, the use of general indices that aggregate multiple features of friendship is limited as it fails to recognize friendship as a process. By distinguishing between interactions and relationships and treating them in a process-oriented way, one can go beyond questions about whether positivity in friendship is good for well-being or not. In the next section we discuss three hypotheses about friendship that are predicated on a structural organization in which interactions precede relationships which, in turn, are related to well-being.

USING A STRUCTURAL APPROACH TO STUDY THE DEVELOPMENT AND THE EFFECTS OF FRIENDSHIP

In this section, we discuss findings from three sets of analyses taken from our ongoing studies. Although each addresses a different question, they share a concern with both features and process. The first project addresses a basic point from Hinde's (1987) model, specifically whether there are increases over time in the relationship measures as a function of initial measures of interactions. The second concerns the path model implied in Hinde's model, specifically that the association between the measures of interactions and measure of well-being will be moderated by relationship measures. The third question we present is built on the first. It asks whether the association between measures of interactions and relationships is stronger among middle-class early adolescents than among those from lower-middle-class or upper-middle-class families. Each of these studies is presented briefly with an emphasis on how the question assesses features of friendship and the association between them.

Are Interactions Antecedent to Relationships?

The first question addresses one of the most basic propositions of Hinde's model, specifically that friendships proceed from interactions to relationships. We chose to study this hypothesized pattern of associations with two waves of data taken from a longitudinal study of friendship conducted with 260 early adolescent girls and boys. At each of two times, separated by a six month interval, measures of interactions, specifically companionship and instrumental aid, and measures of relationships, specifically security and closeness, taken from the *Friendship Qualities Scale* (FQS) (Bukowski et al., 1994) were available for each of the participants in the study. Participants had used the FQS to rate aspects of their interactions and relationship with the peers whom they identified as their best friend. These scores were used to assess a model, shown in Figure 8.1, in which the measures of interaction were identified as being antecedent to the measures of relationship.

The model was tested with a subset (N = 180) of the total sample, specifically those participants who had rated their interaction and relationship

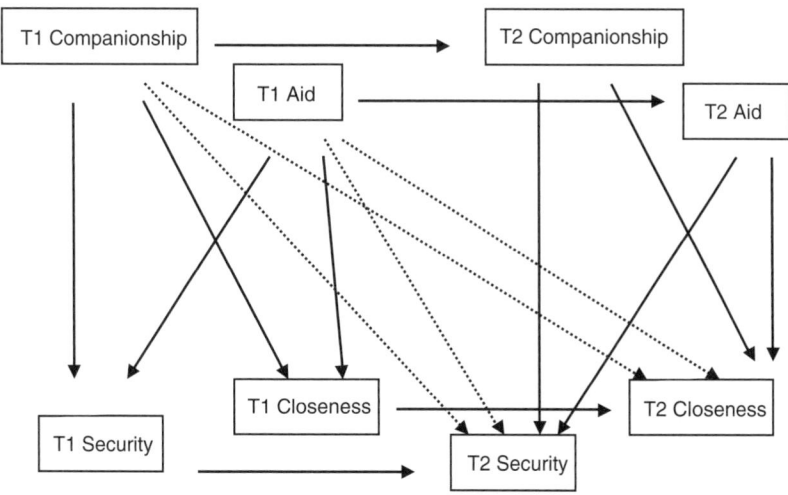

FIGURE 8.1. Measures of interaction with a friend are treated as antecedents of relationship measures.

with the same peer at both times. The critical feature of our model was to assess whether interaction scores at Time 1 would predict scores on the relationship variables six months later at Time 2 after the effects of the relationship measures at Time 1 had been accounted for (in Figure 8.1, these paths are shown as dashed lines). The findings were consistent with the hypotheses based on Hinde's model. Interactions at Time 1 (i.e., measures of companionship and help) were positively associated with the relationship measures at Time 2 (i.e., closeness and security). This pattern shows that high scores on measures of interaction lead to high score on measures of relationship levels at a later time. Beyond confirming the value of taking a process approach to studying the dynamics of friendship during early adolescence, these findings point to the importance of distinguishing between measures of interaction and relationship.

Relationship measures as mediators

The second question is concerned with the presumed flow from interactions to relationships to well-being. We tested this meditational model with the same data used in the previous analysis with the addition of a measure of general self-worth taken from The Perceived Competence Scale for Children (Harter, 1982). This measure was used as the index of well-being. The model we tested is shown in Figure 8.2. The analysis of

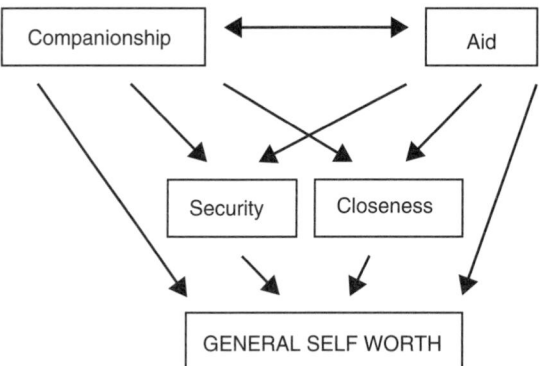

FIGURE 8.2. Relationship measures (i.e., security and closeness) mediate the association between measures of interactions (i.e., aid and companionship) and outcome measure.

this model focused on whether the associations between the interaction measures and the measure of well-being were mediated by the relationship measures. That is, we assessed whether the relationship measures would account for the association between the interaction score and the measure of well-being. Observing this form of mediation would confirm the process implied in Hinde's model in which interactions leads to relations that, in turn, lead to well-being.

Structural equation models provided clear evidence of this mediational process. The observed association between the measures of interaction (i.e., companionship and aid) and the measure of well-being was completely explained by the two relationship measures. The findings confirm that in early adolescence, aspects of relationships, rather than of interaction, carry the significance of friendship. They confirm the process that is at the center of Hinde's model. Specifically they show that measures of interaction are indirectly associated with the measure of well-being via their association with measures of relationships, which are directly related to well-being. These findings do not show that interactions are not important. Instead, their value is as antecedents to relationship features that, in turn, affect outcomes.

Do These Associations between Interactions Vary as a Function Of Risk?

Our third and final question concerns whether the association between interactions and relationships vary as a function of socioeconomic status (SES). Typically, SES-related risk has been treated as a negative linear association.

According to this view, levels of problematic outcomes are seen more frequently among lower-SES girls and boys than among those from upper-SES families. This association has been referred to as the "SES gradient" (Adler & Snibbe, 2003). Recent evidence has challenged this emphasis on linearity (Luthar, 2003). It shows that the association between SES and well-being is best represented by a curve in which problem behaviors tend to be highest among adolescents from either low- or high-SES families and to be lowest among adolescents who are at the centre of the SES spectrum. Our project is concerned with understanding whether the "risk" associated with SES is related to friendship experiences.

Our analysis differs from typical research on risk and SES in two important ways. First, most research on risk assesses whether a particular problematic outcome tends to be higher or lower among individuals at different places along the SES spectrum. That is, it takes an outcome-oriented approach. In contrast, we are interested in variations in the organization between variables as a function of SES. Second, risk research typically focuses on problem behavior per se. Our assessment of risk is concerned with the flow of processes that are presumed to underlie the unfolding of experiences believed to be important for development. That is, our goal was to assess whether the association between measures of interactions and measures of relationships varies as a function of SES. Our analysis assesses both linear and curvilinear variations related to SES in the association between measures of interaction and measures of relationship.

The data for this analysis were taken from a sample of 380 early adolescent (school grades 4, 5, and 6) boys and girls from Barranquilla, a Caribbean city in northern Colombia in Latin America. The participants were from the six levels of the "estratos" that define the official neighborhood-based social status system in Colombia. Each neighborhood in the country is designated at one of the six levels of the system according to several social indicators of its inhabitants and its facilities (e.g., quality of housing). The lowest level is 1 and the highest level is 6. As part of their participation in a larger study, they completed the Network of Relationships Inventory (NRI) (Furman & Buhrmester, 1985). Here we report on the variations in the association between the NRI subscale for companionship, which is a measure of interactions, and the subscale of intimacy, which is a measure of relationship. Our analysis was simple. The measure of intimacy was used as the dependent variable in a multiple regression equation in which there were five predictors. They were the linear and curvilinear effects of SES, the measure of companionship, and the interactions between companionship and

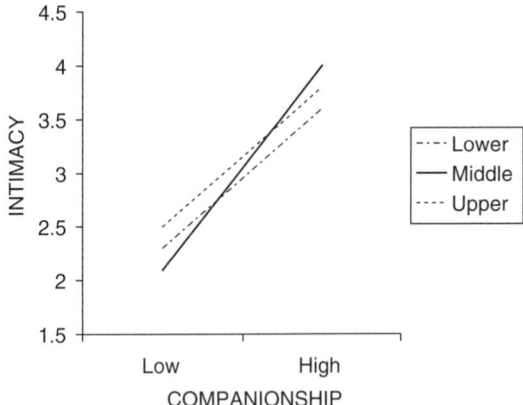

FIGURE 8.3. The association between companionship and intimacy is stronger among early adolescents from middle levels of socioeconomic status, as measured by neighborhood *estrato* index, than among those from either the highest or the lowest groups.

the two SES measures. We were particularly interested in the effects of the latter two predictors. That is, we wanted to know if the association between companionship and intimacy would be moderated by SES and whether this moderation would be linear or nonlinear.

The findings from this analysis are shown in Figure 8.3. The results included significant effects for three of the five predictors, specifically the measure of companionship and the two interactions. The findings indicate the association between companionship and intimacy was stronger for early adolescents from neighborhoods in the middle to upper *estrato* categories (levels 4 and 5) than it was for the upper and lower *estratos*. It was roughly the same for the boys and girls in the lower (levels 1, 2, and 3) and highest (level 6) *estratos* categories. These findings show that the structure between these friendship measures differs for lower, middle, and upper-SES youth.

In one respect, these findings reveal a form of SES-related risk, and in another way they do not. They do not show that friendship intimacy is related to SES in a univariate manner. SES was not associated with intimacy in either a linear or curvilinear manner. Nevertheless, it shows that the process model of friendship where interactions lead to relationships is weaker among early adolescents from the lowest and highest parts of the SES spectrum. At the least, this pattern of findings indicates that the experience of friendship varies as a function of SES, and that upper and lower

SES adolescents share less intimacy with the friends with whom they have the most companionship.

Study Summary

The three sets of findings reported in this section are based on a structural approach to understanding friendship. The three questions addressed basic aspects of Hinde's (1987) model of relationship. Using data taken from early adolescent samples, we showed that (a) earlier indices of interactions positively predicted later measures of relationships; (b) measures of relationship mediate the association between measures of interaction and an index of well-being; and (c) that SES-related variations in the association between interactions and relationships may be one reason that early adolescents from upper and lower SES neighborhoods are more at risk for problematic outcomes than are boys and girls from the upper-middle-class.

SUMMARY

In this chapter, the concepts of representation, structure, and process were used to explore the challenges and opportunities of friendship in early adolescence. It was argued that research on the development of representations of friendship has been more extensive than research on the organization or associations among the many facets that make up friendship. Although children and early adolescents have recognized the multifaceted nature of friendship, researchers have ignored the differences between the particular aspects of friendship and have instead used broad indices of friendship positivity. At least one theory (Hinde, 1987) shows that an understanding of the process of friendship needs to distinguish between its fundamental constituents, specifically aspects of interactions and relationships. An implicit feature of Hinde's model is that research on friendship in early adolescence needs to consider the specific features of friendship and the structure or organization among them. Findings taken from our ongoing studies show the value of using this approach to in research on a central part of life in early adolescence.

ACKNOWLEDGMENTS

Work on this chapter was supported by a grant from the Social Sciences and Humanities Research Council of Canada. The authors are grateful to Dominique Paiement for her careful bibliographic assistance.

REFERENCES

Adler, N.E., & Snibbe, A.C. (2003). The role of psychosocial processes in explaining the gradient between socioeconomic status and health. *Current Directions in Psychological Science, 12,* 119–123.

Adler, T., & Furman, W. (1988). A model for close relationships and relationship dysfunctions. In S.W. Duck (Ed.), *Handbook of personal relationships: theory, research, and interventions.* New York: Wiley.

Aristotle (1973). Nicomachean ethics. In R. McKeon (Ed.) *Introduction to Aristote (2nd Ed.)* Chicago: University of Chicago Press.

Belle, D. (1989). *Children's social networks and social supports.* New York: Wiley.

Berndt, T.J. (1982). The features and effects of friendship in early adolescence. *Child Development, 53,* 1447–1460.

(1986). Children's comments about their friends. In M. Perlmutter (Ed.), *Minnesota symposium on child psychology* (Vol. 18, pp. 189–212). Hillsdale, NJ: Erlbaum.

(2002). Friendship quality and social development. *Current Directions in Psychological Science, 11,* 7–10.

(2004). Children's friendships: Shifts over a half-century in perspectives on their development and their effects. *Merrill-Palmer Quarterly, 50,* 206–223.

(1996). Exploring the effects of friendship quality on social development. In W.M. Bukowski, A.F. Newcomb, and W.W. Hartup (Eds.), *The company they keep: Friendship during childhood and adolescence* (pp. 322–345). New York: Cambridge University Press.

Berndt, T.J., & Perry, T.B. (1986). Children's perceptions of friendships as supportive relationships. *Developmental Psychology, 22,* 640–648.

Bigelow, B.J. (1977). Children's friendship expectations: A cognitive-developmental study. *Child Development, 48,* 246–253.

Blatz, W.E. (1966). *Human Security.* Toronto: University of Toronto Press.

Blum, L. (1980). *Friendship, altruism, and morality.* London: Routledge & Kegan Paul.

Blumer, H. (1969). *Symbolic interactionism: Perspective and method.* Englewood, NJ: Prentice-Hall.

Buhrmester, D. (1990). Intimacy of friendship, interpersonal competence, and adjusment during preadolescence and adolescence. *Child Development, 61,* 1101–1111.

Buhrmester, D., & Furman, W. (1987). The development of companionship and intimacy. *Child Development, 58,* 1101–1113.

Bukowski, W.M., Brendgen, M., & Vitaro, F. (2007). Peers and Socialization: Effects on Externalizing and Internalizing Problems. In J.E. Grusec and P.D. Hastings (Eds.), *Handbook of socialization: Theory and research* (pp. 355–381). New York: Guilford.

Bukowski, W.M., Hoza, B., & Boivin, M. (1994). Measuring friendship quality during pre- and early adolescence: The development and psychometric properties of the friendship qualities scale. *Journal of Social and Personal Relationships, 11,* 471–484.

Bukowski, W.M., Motzoi, C., & Meyer, F. (2009). Friendship as process, function, and outcome. In K. Rubin, W.M. Bukowski and B. Laursen (Eds.), *Handbook of peer interactions, relationships, and groups* (pp. 217–231). New York: Guilford.

Bukowski, W.M., Newcomb, A.F., & Hoza, B. (1987). Friendship conceptions among early adolescents: A longitudinal study of stability and change. *Journal of Early Adolescence, 7*, 143–152.

Bukowski, W.M., & Sippola, L.K. (1996). Friendship and morality: (How) are they related? In W.M. Bukowski, A.F. Newcomb, & W.W. Hartup (Eds.), *The company they keep: Friendship during childhood and adolescence* (pp. 238–261). New York: Cambridge University Press.

(2005). Friendship and development: Putting the most human relationship in its place. In R. Larson and L. Jensen (Eds.), *New directions for child and adolescent development* (pp. 91–98). SanFrancisco: Jossey-Bass.

Coleman, J. (1974). *Relationships in adolescence.* London: Routledge & Kegan Paul.

Cooley, C.H. (1964). *Human nature and the social order.* New York: Academic Press.

(1909). *Social organization.* New York: Scribner's.

Davies, B. (1982). *Life in the classroom and playground.* London: Routledge & Kegan Paul.

Demir, M., & Urberg, K.A. (2004). Friendship and adjustment among adolescents. *Journal of Experimental Child Psychology, 88*, 68–82.

Douvan, E., & Adelson, J. (1966). *The adolescent experience.* New York: Wiley.

Eichhorn, D. (1980). The school. In M. Johnson (Ed.) *Toward adolescence: The middle school years* (pp. 56–73). Chicago: National Society for the Study of Education.

Fine, G.A. (1981). Friends, impression management, and preadolescent behavior. In S.R. Asher & J.M. Gottman (Eds.), *The development of children's friendships* (pp. 29–52). New York : Cambridge University Press.

Friedman, M. (1989). Friendship and moral growth. *The Journal of Value Inquiry, 23*, 3–13.

Furman, W., & Buhrmester, D. (1985). Children's perceptions of the personal relationships in their social networks. *Developmental Psychology, 21*, 1016–1024.

Furman, W., & Robbins, P. (1985). What's the point? Issues in the selection of treatment objectives. In B.H. Schneider, K.H. Rubin, & J.E. Ledingham (Eds.). *Children's peer relations: Issues in assessment and intervention* (pp. 41–54). New York: Springer-Verlag.

Gauze, C., Bukowski, W.M., Aquan-Assee, J., & Sippola, L.K. (1996). Interactions between family environment and friendship and associations with self-perceived well-being during early adolescence. *Child Development, 67*, 2201–2216.

Gottman, J.M. (1983). How children become friends. *Monographs of the Society for Research in Child Development, 48*, (3, Serial No. 201).

Harter, S. (1982). The perceived competence scale for children. *Child Development, 53*, 87–97.

Hartup, W.W. (1979). Two worlds of childhood. *American Psychologist, 34*, 944–950.

Hartup, W.W., Larsen, B., Stewart, M.I., & Easterson, A. (1988). Conflict and the friendship relation of young children. *Child Development, 59*, 1590–1600.

Hartup, W.W., & Stevens, N. (1997). Friendships and adaptation in the life course. *Psychological Bulletin, 121*, 355–370.

Hinde, R.A. (1979). *Towards understanding relationships.* New York: Academic Press.

(1987). *Individuals, relationships and culture*. Cambridge: Cambridge University Press.

Hodges, E.V.E., Mallone, M.J., & Perry, D.G. (1997). Individual risk and social risk as interacting determinants of victimization in the peer group. *Developmental Psychology, 33*, 1032–1039.

Luthar, S. S. (2003). The culture of affluence: The psychological costs of material wealth. *Child Development, 74*, 1581–1593.

Mannarino, A. P. (1978). Friendship patterns and self-concept development in pre-adolescent males. *Journal of Genetic Psychology, 133*, 105–110.

Mead, G.H. (1934). *Mind, self, and society*. Chicago: University of Chicago Press.

Newcomb, A., & Bagwell, C. (1995). Children's friendship relations: A meta-analytic review. *Psychological Bulletin, 117*, 306–347.

Newcomb, A.F., & Brady, J.E. (1982). Mutuality in boys' friendship relations. *Child Development, 53*, 392–395.

Peevers, B.H., & Secord, P.F. (1973). Developmental changes in attribution of descriptive concepts to persons. *Journal of Personality and Social Psychology, 27*, 120–128.

Pinto, G., Bombi, A.S., & Cordioli, A. (1997). Similarity of friends in three countries: A study of children's drawings. *International Journal of Behavioral Development, 20*, 453–469.

Raymond, J. (1986). *A passion for friends*. Boston: Beacon.

Rizzo, T. A. (1989). *Friendship development among children in school*. Norwood, NJ: Ablex.

Rubin, K.H., Bukowski, W., & Parker, J.G. (1998). Peer interactions, relationships, and groups. In N. Eisenberg (Ed.) & W. Damon (Series Ed.), *Handbook of child psychology: Vol. 3. Social, emotional, and personality development* (5th ed., pp. 619–700). New York: Wiley.

Rubin, K.H., Bukowski, W.M., & Parker, J.G. (2006). Peer interactions, relationships and groups. In W. Damon (Series Ed.) and N. Eisenberg (Volume Ed.), *The handbook of child psychology* (6th Edition, pp. 571–645). New York: Wiley.

Rutter, M. (1989). Pathways from childhood to adult life. *Journal of Child Psychology and Psychiatry and Allied Disciplines, 30*, 23–51.

Salter (Ainsworth), Mary, D. (1940). The concept of security as a basis for the evaluation of adjustment based on the concept of security. *Child development series, 18*. Toronto: University of Toronto Press.

Selman, R. L. (1981). The child as a friendship philosopher. In S. R. Asher & J. M. Gottman (Eds.), *The development of children's friendships* (pp. 242–272). New York: Cambridge University Press.

Shantz, C.U., & Shantz D.W. (1985). Conflict between children: Social-cognitive and sociometric correlates. In M.W. Berkowitz (Ed.), *New directions for child development: Vol. 7. Peer conflict and psychological growth* (pp. 3–21). San Francisco: Jossy-Bass.

Shantz, C.U. (1987). Conflicts between children. *Child Development, 58*, 283–305.

Shantz, D.W. (1986). Conflict, aggression, and peer status: An observational study. *Child Development, 57*, 1322–1332.

Smoller, J., & Youniss, J. (1982). Social development through friendship. In K. H. Rubin & H. S. Ross (Eds.), *Peer relationships and social skills in childhood* (pp. 277–298). New York: Springer-Verlag.

Strough, J., Swenson, L.M., & Cheng, S. (2001) Friendship, gender and preadolescents' representation of peer collaboration. *Merrill-Palmer Quarterly, 47,* 475–499.

Sullivan, H.S. (1953). *The interpersonal theory of psychiatry.* New York: Norton.

Weiss, R.S. (1974). The provisions of social relationships. In Z. Rubin (Ed.), *Doing unto others.* Englewood Cliffs, NJ: Prentice-Hall.

Youniss, J. (1980). *Parents and peers in social development: A Sullivan-Piaget perspective.* Chicago: University of Chicago Press.

9

Schools, Peers, and the Big Picture
of Adolescent Development

ROBERT CROSNOE

University of Texas At Austin

The pioneering work of Jean Piaget is now so closely identified with psychology that the fact he held appointments in sociology and wrote sociology texts is often forgotten – by both psychologists and sociologists. This trend is unfortunate because Piaget's approach to human development serves as a meeting point – and integration point – between these two disciplines as well as others so crucial to building a scientific base of understanding about adolescence. After all, Piaget's constructivist perspective emphasizes the give-and-take between developing youth and their environments, between the personal and the social. This give-and-take can best be deconstructed, therefore, by drawing on the real strengths of both of these two disciplines as well as other related disciplines.

As a trained sociologist and social demographer whose home base and primary audience has steadily moved toward developmental psychology, I have drawn heavily on developmental insights to understand the contextual and structural conditions of society. Specifically, in my work, I examine population trends and societal inequalities as manifested in the American educational system but try to view them through the more intimate lens of developmental and interpersonal process. Basically, my stance is that a population looks they way it does, in part, because of the normative patterns and group differences in how young people in that population grow up and find their places in the world. This idea underlies my somewhat Piagetian working conceptual model of adolescent development. In this model, development unfolds within a field of constraints imposed by the environment but is also acted on by the developing adolescent, with environment referring not just to the commonly studied proximal settings of

The research in this chapter is based on Robert Crosnoe, Fitting In, Standing Out: Navigating the Social Challenges of High School to Get an Education (Cambridge, 2011).

the developmental ecology (e.g., the family, peer group, neighborhood), but also to the larger pieces of the very machinery of society – organizations, institutions, stratification systems, culture, and even history itself.

Working from this conceptual model, I have come to realize how true it is that no single discipline can do justice to all sides of the cross-level transactional processes at the heart of adolescent development. Consequently, social and behavioral scientists from diverse disciplines have to make up the difference in trying to construct a complete picture of adolescent development. They can do so by talking to each other, sharing with each other, and, eventually, internalizing each others' perspectives as background music in their heads as they work along their own disciplinary paths. In that spirit, this chapter is intended to provide some background music to developmentalists from a more psychological orientation as they go about doing what they do to elucidate the vulnerabilities and opportunities that adolescents face in modern society. To do so, I discuss both general and specific ways in which high schools serve as contexts of adolescent development in the United States and how this role of high schools is embedded in a set of converging macro-level trends.

This discussion draws on past work by psychologists, sociologists, and other social and behavioral scientists as well as my own work over the last decade – quantitative analyses of a nationally representative sample of nearly 8,000 American high school students who participated in three years of data collection as part of the National Longitudinal Study of Adolescent Health (Add Health; see Harris, 2008), as well as qualitative analyses of a smaller sample of thirty-two students at a single diverse public high school (Lamar) in Texas. Worth stressing is that there is a great deal of variability – by race/ethnicity, immigration status, social class – in the patterns and processes discussed in this chapter, variability that is caused by and contributes to societal inequality. Of these various forms of social stratification, however, the clearest dividing line for this topic is gender.

THE SOCIAL AND ACADEMIC SIDES OF SCHOOL

As a starting point, decades of developmentally informed research on education has resulted in a broad consensus that the social dynamics of high school life affect the academic prospects of American adolescents. This consensus is built on some classic studies, *The Adolescent Society* (Coleman, 1961) most prominently. It is reflected in a host of groundbreaking examinations of adolescent school-based peer crowds – nerds, jocks, goths, and so forth – and the academic implications of membership in such crowds from psychologists (Barber, Eccles, & Stone, 2001; Klute & Brown, 2003), linguists (Eckert, 1989), sociologists (Kinney, 1999; Milner, 2004), economists (Akerlof & Kranton, 2002), and multidisciplinary teams (Steinberg, Brown, & Dornbusch, 1996). It is also illustrated by constructivist investigations of how middle and high school peer dynamics serve as a conduit for the production and reproduction of culture and inequality in ways that also affect education (Adler & Adler, 1998; Carter, 2006; Eder, Parker, & Evans, 1995).

At the heart of all of this work is the recognition that high schools serve two major roles in American society, one official and sanctioned and the other much less so, although no less powerful (Labaree, 1997). On the one hand, high school is an *educational institution*, and, as such, a place where curricula and instruction are delivered to students charged with learning and skill acquisition. This institutional role of high school aligns with the long-standing and widely held cultural belief about the manifest function of schools in society, which is to promote economic productivity and civic stability (Lee, Smith, & Croninger, 1997; Schneider, 2007). On the other hand, high school is also a *social context* in which young people are brought together for long periods of time each day across many years and, in the process, construct networks of social relations and related systems of norms, values, customs, and rituals. This social role of high school does not map onto the official mission of the educational system but affects adolescents' life trajectories just the same and, importantly, can both promote and hinder schools' attempts to follow that official mission (Eccles & Barber, 1999; Frank et al., 2008; McFarland & Pals, 2005).

Adult stakeholders in the educational system – parents, teachers, and policy makers to name three – tend to view high schools primarily through the institutional lens. Partly, this reflects their understanding of the importance of the high school career to adolescents' future socioeconomic attainment and, therefore, the need for schools to serve adolescents effectively and for adolescents to get the most academically from their schools. At the same time, this common adult view also reflects how far removed most adults are from their own high school lives. With years of distance from high school, many have lost touch with the immediacy of the social currents that play out with great frequency and intensity within high schools.

For adolescents, the story is quite different. Still caught up in those very same social currents, they tend to emphasize the noninstitutional role of high school (Johnson, Crosnoe, & Elder, 2001; Lightfoot, 1983; Milner, 2004). Indeed, the adolescents I interviewed at Lamar almost universally defined the high school experience in terms of relationships formed and maintained at high school rather than through more academic pursuits. For example, a tenth-grade Latina made a clear distinction between what high school is "supposed to be" (academic) and what it is (social). As another example, a ninth-grade European-American boy explained that, at its core, high school is just "a big building with lots of people in it."

Of course, rather than an educational institution *or* a social context, high schools are *both*. These two sides of school are inextricably intertwined, and, as result, understanding adolescent development and secondary education requires a consideration of this interplay.

Connecting the Two Sides of High School

This interplay between the social and academic sides of high school is bidirectional. What goes on in the social side affects what goes on in the academic side, and vice versa. Given space constraints, I focus on only one direction here. As previously noted, the social dynamics of high schools have implications for adolescents' learning and academic achievement. Integrating the insights of past research on adolescent development, education, and the connection between the two from across multiple disciplines of social and behavioral science, my general conclusion is that the academic significance of the social side of schooling is channeled through adolescents' own personal socioemotional development.

Starting with the *first piece of this pathway*, there are at least three general mechanisms that link the social dynamics of high school to adolescents' personal development. All three are rooted in a developmental reality; namely that because of the evolving neurological makeup of adolescents and their psychological need to establish themselves independently from parents, young people become highly social creatures during the high school years. Not only do they have a strong need for social connections, as all humans do, but they also draw more heavily than children or adults on their social relationships, groups, and networks in understanding themselves and the world (Furstenberg, 2000; Guyer, McClure-Tone, Shiffrin, Pine, & Nelson, 2009; Steinberg, 2008).

One mechanism linking the social dynamics of high school to adolescents' personal development is that high schools are a major setting in which adolescents are socialized into prevailing norms. Echoing *The Adolescent Society*, high schools are their own cultures, where young people learn what and who is valued. This socialization does not necessarily compete with socialization at home or church or in other settings, but sometimes it does (Allen, Porter, McFarland, Marsh, & McElhaney, 2005; Steinberg, 2001). For example, the prevailing norms in the student body of Lamar generally support academic achievement and, even more so, college going. This normative structure, which cuts across most segments of the student body, is a conventional stance in line with what many adults view as important. Yet, prevailing norms also widely support substance use as a form of social achievement, which is a stance more oppositional to conventional adult norms. These two dimensions of peer culture at Lamar converge to serve as a set of standards, which many adolescents will internalize when navigating themselves through this peer culture.

Another mechanism is that high schools are opportunity structures for behavior, helping determine whether adolescents will engage in behaviors in line with or against their own inclinations, motivations, and desires. The more prevalent a behavior is among students in a high school, the more likely any one student will transition into that behavior over time. This phenomenon is not simply a result of modeling or socialization. It reflects the greater ease with which an adolescent can select into or be drawn into a behavior when surrounded by others who are doing it (Bearman & Bruckner, 2001; Crosnoe, Frank, & Muller, 2004). Going back to Lamar as an example, substance use requires more than the desire to use. It is greatly facilitated by knowledge about how to obtain alcohol or drugs illegally and how to use them without being caught, knowledge that is more likely to be accessed by adolescents attending a school like Lamar than by similarly inclined adolescents attending a high school in which substance use is less prevalent. Again, opportunity can act independently of personal disposition.

A third mechanism linking the social dynamics of high school to adolescents' personal development is that high school peers collectively provide the reference group that adolescents need for self-assessment (McFarland & Pals, 2005; Sandstrom, Cillessen, & Eisenhower, 2003). By comparing themselves to others in their high school and by studying the reactions they receive from others at school and the status they seem to have at school, adolescents work their way through the developmental task of understanding who they are and what their place is in the world (Kinney, 1999; Roesser & Eccles, 2000). In Lamar, for example, adolescents found it next to impossible to assess their own social competence without using others at their school as a benchmark. They were constantly measuring themselves against the backdrop of school peers and interpreting their own lives through the prism of what was valued in their own peer groups and in the school as a whole.

The takeaway message of all three of these mechanisms is the same. Where adolescents attend high school matters to a full range of behaviors, conditions, and characteristics that are encapsulated in development.

Starting with the *second piece of this pathway*, there are at least two general mechanisms that link adolescents' within-school personal development to their academic progress. Both are predicated on the idea that learning and academic achievement are rooted in more than intellectual competencies. Instead, academic progress is a multidetermined phenomenon, in which noncognitive factors can undermine or magnify cognitive skills, helping some adolescents achieve at or above their skill levels and pushing other adolescents towards underachievement (Eccles & Wigfield, 2002).

The first of these two mechanisms linking adolescents' within-school personal development and their academic progress is that the personal and social identities that adolescents develop within their high schools can fall anywhere along the distribution from antischool to proschool. In other words, some adolescents may develop antischool postures that cause them to devalue the widely shared aims of school and, as a result, disengage from the educational process. Even intellectually able adolescents may experience academic failures if their orientation toward school prevents them from fully capitalizing on what school has to offer them. Alternatively, less academically capable adolescents may do far better than expected if their orientation toward school keeps them motivated and effortful (Carter, 2006; Weinstein, 2002). This mechanism is rooted in the kinds of peer values that adolescents are exposed to at school.

The second of these two mechanisms linking adolescents' within-school personal development and their academic progress is that the very process of navigating the social side of high school can be hard work (Allen et al., 2005). To the extent that adolescents can become preoccupied with this social work, they may be distracted from their academic pursuits and responsibilities (Eder et al., 1995; McFarland & Pals, 2005). Importantly, this mechanism is more independent of the substance of peer values in a high school. Consider an adolescent who, in trying to maintain social status in an academically oriented high school with a long tradition of sending graduates to college, joins many clubs and commits to multiple activities. At the same time, consider an adolescent who, in trying to maintain social status in a high school with a vibrant party scene, attends many social events and dates frequently. Both of these adolescents may be preoccupied and distracted by these efforts in ways that reduce the translation of their potential ability into their actual achievement.

These two mechanisms linking adolescents' within-school personal development and their academic progress were summed up for me by a tenth-grade European-American girl at Lamar who discussed the struggle she sometimes felt pursuing *both* social and academic achievement at Lamar. She drew on a lesson she had learned in world history class about how many World War II–era German citizens did not rise up against the Holocaust, explaining that, if one hears that the sky is green long enough, she might come to see that the sky is green rather than blue and then act accordingly. This young woman understood that some adolescents were at risk academically because they came to see that the sky was green (e.g., achievement did not matter), whereas others were at risk because they sometimes forgot that sky was *not* green because they had too much else to worry about at school.

Linking together all pieces of the pathway (social dynamics→ personal development→ academic progress), then, suggests that high school is where young people are exposed to instruction and curriculum but also where they are exposed to a social system that, by affecting the kinds of adolescents they come to be, has implications for how they approach and engage with these academic resources. Whether a high school is good or bad, therefore, depends on more than its course offerings, funding, and teacher credentials. The degree to which it serves as a safe, healthy place to come of age is also important.

HISTORICAL PERSPECTIVE

If, as decades of social and behavioral research and theory suggest, the academic consequences of adolescents' search for themselves amid the contradictory messages of high school peer cultures have been around a long time (Brumberg, 1997; Coleman, 1961; Modell, 1989), then these consequences are likely well known to most adults with some stake in the education of young people now, such as parents and teachers. Yet, just because this connection between the social and academic sides of high school is a long-standing one does not mean that the nature and implications of it are historically stable. Indeed, a careful inspection of macro-level trends suggests that, as we move into the new century, this connection likely operates in different ways and means vastly different things for adolescence and the transition to adulthood. I want to focus on four such trends here as a context for understanding the discussion laid out above within the current historical moment.

Dramatic Changes in U.S. Demography

When Coleman published *The Adolescent Society* in 1961, the American high school population stood at about nine million adolescents. Today, it is approaching 20 million (U.S. Census Bureau, 2007). In fact, we are currently witnessing the largest high school graduating classes ever. Partly, these peaks in high school enrolment are carryover effects from the Baby Boom generation. In other words, today's large high school cohort is made up of the children of the large high school cohorts of the 1960s and 1970s. Yet, more than cohort reproduction is at work here. In particular, the reform of federal immigration laws in the 1960s restored the size of immigration flows to levels not seen since early in the twentieth century (Zhou, 1997). Given the increased diversity of this contemporary immigration stream by national origin, today's high school cohort is not only the biggest it has ever been but also the most racially and ethnically heterogeneous it has ever been (Hernandez, Denton, & Macartney, 2007). For example, in thirty years, European Americans have gone from an overwhelming majority of the youth population of the United States to a bare majority (U.S. Census Bureau, 2007).

With this demographic trend in mind, the well-documented patterns that adolescents feel a greater sense of belonging in small, homogenous high schools and that they perform better academically when they feel a greater sense of belonging in school seem to be out of sync with the new reality of secondary education in the United States (Goldsmith, 2004; Johnson et al., 2001; McNeely, Nonnemaker, & Blum, 2002;). As a result, the growth and diversification of the high school student population likely means that finding one's place in the social systems of high schools is more difficult and requires more work.

School Reorganization

For a variety of reasons, including the widely held public perception that the American educational system is falling behind its counterparts in other industrialized nations (National Academy of Sciences, 2007), a proliferation of school reforms in recent decades have resulted in what is often referred to as the Shopping Mall High School (Powell, Farrar, & Cohen, 1985). In short, high school curricula are now characterized by an abundance of choice, with students facing an increasing number of options about what courses to take, at what level, and when as they move from grade to grade. This trend means that incoming freshmen can take a multitude of pathways through the curriculum in the ensuing years they are in high school. Some of these pathways position adolescents for entry into elite colleges, and others lead to dead ends and dropout (Lee et al., 1997; Schneider, 2007). In addition, the implementation of the No Child Left Behind law earlier this decade has created performance pressures on the school and staff levels that trickle down to adolescents, with the entire school punished or rewarded for students' rankings on academic benchmarks (Darling-Hammond, 2006).

In many ways, these school reforms represent a positive trend, but empirical evidence from sociologists of education suggest that they also carry hidden risks. For example, adolescents from more socioeconomically advantaged backgrounds are better able to draw on the pools of social and cultural capital that their family statuses provide them to navigate increasingly differentiated, optional curricula in ways that give them a major competitive edge. As another example, the cumulative nature of curricular pathways means that early academic actions and decisions can become highly self-propagating. These two hidden risks are, of course, related (Attewell & Thurston, 2008; Morgan, 2005). In this climate, navigating the high school curriculum is a high-stakes game on an uneven playing field, in which any one misstep – such as an academic misstep caused by social problems – is hard to undo.

The Information Technology Revolution

The technological advances of the last two decades as well as the democratization of both wired and wireless communication are transforming high schools in general and adolescents' social lives in particular. Adolescents communicate with teachers, do homework, and study online, and they connect to each other through email, texting, IM, social networking sites (e.g., Facebook, Twitter), and cell phones (Brown, Green, & Harper, 2002; Greenfield & Yan, 2006). Indeed, according to the Pew Internet and American Life Project, a larger majority of adolescents use all of these means of communication on a regular basis (Lenhart, 2008). As a result, the social worlds of adolescents are becoming larger and more diffuse yet also more ambiguous. On the one hand, the Internet allows adolescents to identify and connect to other people like them, regardless of place, and to find a community of their own. On the other hand, it has a layer of anonymity that can pose dangers to young people (Kraut, Patterson, Lundmark, Kiesler, Muhopadhyay, & Scherlis, 1998; Suzuki & Calzo, 2004). In Lamar, for example, just about every girl I interviewed used social networking sites to maintain relationships with other youth outside of their school but also had experience as a target of online aggression from someone at school or knew someone who had such experience.

The implications of this technological revolution for the connection between the social and academic sides of high school is somewhat paradoxical. Adolescents having academically troubling social problems in high school have, at once, more opportunities to find alternate arenas of social belonging and connection but also less opportunity to escape the reach of their high school social arenas.

Economic Restructuring

A final trend to consider is the large-scale restructuring of the American economy since the early 1970s. Basically, the manufacturing sector of the traditional industrial economy has been shrinking while the information/ service sector of the postindustrial economy has been growing. The result is an hourglass shaped labor market in which few options are left between well-paying, stable, professional occupations and low-paying, insecure service jobs (Bernhardt, Morris, Handcock, & Scott, 2001; Goldin & Goldin, 2008). This reshaping of the labor market, in turn, has powerful implications for the educational system. In the past, finding a "good" job with only a high school education – in the automobile industry, for example – and using this job to secure a place in the middle class and/or become upwardly mobile was far more likely than it is today. Consequently, the lifelong returns to college education are at an all-time high (Fischer & Hout, 2006). For example, Census data reveal that the earnings premium for a bachelor's degree versus a high school diploma among men has risen from less than 20 percent to almost 70 percent in the last thirty years (Baum & Ma, 2007). Given the link between income and many other life course trajectories, including marriage and health (McLanahan, 2004; Mirowsky & Ross, 2003), this trend is not just about money.

How does economic restructuring of this kind relate to the connection between the social and academic sides of high school? By raising the critical nature of college education for the life course, economic restructuring has greatly intensified the potential long-term consequences of social problems in high school that filter into the academic domain.

Converging Trends

The changing demography, school organization, technology use, and economic prospects that have characterized recent decades are all realities of contemporary adolescence. As such, they provide the context in which the long-standing connection between the social dynamics of high schools and adolescents' academic fortunes plays out. Compared to their parents and other adults who oversee their educational careers, contemporary adolescents experience this connection in larger, competitive, digitized, and unbounded high schools that pose greater risks and rewards for their futures. Thus, embedding a proximal environmental/developmental process within these distal population-level forces suggests that the social worlds of high schools have effects on young people in and out of school in the short term that can shape their lives in the long term. If so, then the long-standing connection between the social and academic sides of high school is growing more intense. As a result, educational policy that does not recognize this developmental phenomenon – in other words, that focuses too much on the

institutional side of school without paying attention to the potentially coun-
terbalancing social dynamics in school – is unlikely to fulfill all of its goals.

A SPECIFIC DIMENSION OF THE CONNECTION BETWEEN
SOCIAL AND ACADEMIC EXPERIENCES

The connection between the social dynamics in high school and the academic progress of high school students plays out in many varied ways,
some positive and some negative. One way to see how this connection
can undermine the educational mission of high schools and related educational policies is to look at a specific group of adolescents who may be at
risk academically regardless of their academic potential. In other words,
some adolescents may run into academic problems strictly because of
what is going on socially in their high schools. Here, I focus on whether
and how strong social stigma in American society can seep into the high
school and jeopardize the academic prospects of some adolescents relative
to others.

In American youth culture, some characteristic or attribute may be generally stigmatized. As such, adolescents with that characteristics or attribute may
face higher probabilities of being socially marginalized. They face a greater
burden of proof in social situations, having to prove their social worth to others as a way of making up for whatever it is about them that carries a stigma. Of
course, no characteristic is stigmatized everywhere, and some adolescents may
not be stigmatized even if they have a characteristic that is generally stigmatized (Hegerty, 2009; Link & Phelan, 2001). For the most part, however, when
a stigma exists in some context or setting, it raises social risks.

Following Goffman's (1963) classic framework of stigma, two of the most
common ways that individuals are stigmatized is through certain aspects
of physical appearance and through their "tribal" memberships. Obesity is
one of the most prominent examples of appearance-based stigma (Crandall,
1994; Puhl & Brownell, 2001). Family poverty locates young people in a
certain segment of the population that has expectations, status, and value
judgments attached to it (McLoyd, 1998), thereby mapping onto Goffman's
idea of tribal stigma. Importantly, these two types of stigma differ on the
dimensions of visibility – whereas obesity is immediately apparent to
others, poverty is less so. To the extent that adolescents who are obese and/
or come from poor families are socially marginalized in high school in ways
that disrupt their educational trajectories, then, they will illustrate how the
social and academic sides of contemporary U.S. high schools can work at
cross-purposes with each other.

Stigma, Coping, and Consequences

To understand how obese and/or poor youth may be at risk for truncated rates of educational attainment, consider how unpleasant stigmatization can be. When a member of a stigmatized group, adolescents are under a threat of social exclusion and, as a result, often have to work harder to achieve social acceptance or status – all during a developmental stage in which the need for social approval and the pain of social exclusion peaks (La Greca & Lopez, 1998; Sandstrom et al., 2003). Because adolescents are also quite agentic, meaning that they tend to view their lives as under their control, they are motivated to change unpleasant situations, to get themselves out of trouble (Bandura, 2001; Elder, 1998). Some of these attempts to cope with what is happening to them may be positive, others negative. I will get to the former shortly but concentrate on more problematic coping responses for the moment.

Among these more problematic responses to stigmatization and social marginalization are: 1) internalizing the pain of stigma by adjusting self-concepts so that they are consistent with real or perceived external judgments of the self; 2) self-medicating to numb the pain of stigmatization by engaging in different forms of substance use; and 3) avoiding the pain of stigmatization by removing oneself from the site in which stigmatization is occurring (e.g., the high school) or by reducing the importance or value placed on that site (Dance, 2002; Hussong et al., 2001; Yeung & Martin, 2003). In the short term, such coping responses may be perfectly rational, in the sense that they provide momentary relief from social troubles. The long-term implications, however, can be disastrous. We can see how short-term fixes create long-term problems by looking at what, in most racial/ethnic groups and social classes, is seen as the desired transition from high school – enrolling in college (Schneider, 2007). For example, my prior work with Add Health has shown that negative self-concept, alcohol use, and truancy – which map onto internalization, self-medication, and disengagement, respectively – can interfere with adolescents' pathways into college (Crosnoe, 2006; Crosnoe et al., 2004), which, in turn, affect earnings, health, family formation, and other life course trajectories (Fischer & Hout, 2006; Mirowsky & Ross, 2003).

Thus, even if the social problems related to being obese and/or poor in high school are temporary and confined only to the high school period, adolescents may cope with these problems during high school in ways that set into motion a sequential chain of negative events and experiences that extend well beyond high school.

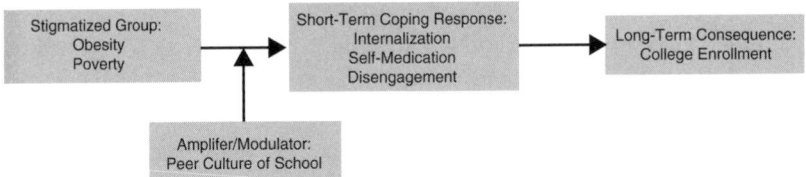

FIGURE 9.1. A blueprint for the disruption of difference.

One final point of consideration is that even the most generalized stigma may be highly variable across local settings (Ross, 1994). The level and intensity of a general stigma that young people encounter in their local settings, then, may determine how they experience that stigma. As a result, the specific social values about body size and money in any one school can amp up or dial down the potential of obesity and poverty to translate into social and then academic problems over time.

Pulling together all of these different strands of thought points to a specific application of the connection between the social and academic sides of high school that I refer to as the Disruption of Difference (see Figure 9.1). In this model, obese and/or poor youth are viewed as different by others in school, and they attempt to cope with this experience of difference in ways that ultimately disrupt their college going, especially in schools in which obesity and poverty are least likely to be found.

To test this model on a national scale, I conducted a series of analyses in which the odds of young people in Add Health enrolling in a four-year college in the four to five years following high school were predicted by a host of adolescent factors measured while they were in high school, including obesity (defined by being at or above the 95th percentile of body mass index for age and gender; see Centers for Disease Control and Prevention, 2000) and family poverty (defined by annual income at or below the federal poverty line; see U.S. Census Bureau, 2009), as well as numerous aspects of developmental stage (e.g., grade, age), demographic location (e.g., race/ethnicity, immigration status), family background (e.g., parent education, family living arrangements), cognitive development (e.g., standardized cognitive test scores), more objective social position (e.g., number of friends, dating activity), and school location (e.g., sector, size, composition). Reflecting my background in social demography, I paid special attention when conducting these analyses to issues of causal inference by utilizing propensity scores (to control for the impact of confounds that could be readily observed) and a class of robustness indices (to gauge the potential impact of confounds that were more difficult to identify and measure).

Obesity and Poverty

Overall, obese girls had 80 percent lower odds of attending high school than nonobese girls with the same race/ethnicity, socioeconomic status, and many other social, academic, family, and school characteristics. This discrepancy in college going, however, varied depending on the average body size of all female students in any given high school. For example, it was significantly larger among girls in high schools in which the average female body size among students was one standard deviation above the national average, and it was significantly smaller in high schools in which the average female body size among students was one standard deviation above the national average. In sum, obese girls in Add Health were much less likely to attend college than otherwise similar nonobese girls, especially in high schools in which obese girls were relatively rare.

To better understand why this might be happening, I added to these analyses measures tapping increases in internalization, self-medication, and disengagement across a two-year period of high school after obesity was measured. In particular, I was interested in how taking these three sets of socioemotional factors into account would attenuate the previously observed "effect" of obesity on college enrollment. Doing so suggested that about one-third of this educational risk of obesity was accounted for by obese girls' higher rates of self-rejection, perceived social isolation, depression (in "thin" schools only), and dislike of school (especially in "thin" schools). In line with the Disruption of Difference, obese girls appeared to be internalizing the stigmatization of school and disengaging from the school setting of this stigmatization, both of which posed risks to their educational trajectories out of high school.

The story was quite different for boys. Reflecting that the stigmatization of obesity is not solely confined to girls, the teenage boys in Add Health also appeared to experience obesity during their high school years in extremely negative ways. For example, obese boys had higher rates of perceived social isolation, academic failure, and disliking school. Nevertheless, despite obese boys' deteriorating social and emotional adjustment during high school, they were not less (or more) likely than nonobese boys to attend college after high school. Moreover, neither the socioemotional profile nor college-going rates of obese boys varied across high schools differing in terms of the average body size of male students.

Turning to poverty, growing up poor can interfere with educational trajectories in a variety of ways, many of which have nothing to do with social stigma or peer relations (Duncan, Brooks-Gunn, Yeung, & Smith, 1998; McLoyd, 1998). Thus, merely showing a link between poverty in high school and college enrollment after high school does not amount to the Disruption of Difference. Instead, to capture the Disruption of Difference, we need to see that this link gets stronger as the *mismatch* between the socioeconomic circumstances of the adolescent and the socioeconomic circumstances of the student body of her/his high school increases. Furthermore, we need to see that the strengthening of this link in situations of adolescent-school mismatch is due to the deteriorating social and emotional adjustment of poor adolescents in these situations.

Not surprisingly, girls whose families fell below the federal poverty line had far lower odds of attending college after high school than otherwise similar nonpoor girls. This gap, however, fluctuated across schools in one important way. In schools in which the majority of the student body had college-educated parents, poor girls had 80 percent lower odds of attending college than nonpoor girls. In schools in which only a small minority of girls came from such socioeconomically advantaged families, these odds were only 60 percent lower. Thus, echoing the basic pattern for obesity, the more the poor girls were part of the mainstream, the better they did. Furthermore, one-fifth of this link between family poverty and college going among girls occurred because poor girls in schools in which the norm among students was to have well-educated parents posted bigger increases in depression and truancy from year to year. In other words, they were unhappy, and they skipped out of attending school.

As expected, boys from poor families also had lower rates of college going after high school. Yet, whether they went to college or not was unrelated to the socioeconomic composition of their schools. Thus, even though poor boys had social and emotional problems, I cannot say for sure whether these problems arose because of the stigma of being different or from many of the other stressful experiences associated with growing up poor.

In sum, the Disruption of Difference offers an example of how the social side of schooling can create problems for the academic side of school that have long-term consequences – but only for girls. In some sense, this was to be expected, considering evidence that girls tend to care more about issues of social integration and exclusion than boys (Rudolph & Conley, 2005). Yet, recall that both girls and boys showed signs that experiencing difference in high school was socially and emotionally difficult. The primary gender difference was that such social and emotional difficulty only disrupted the college going of girls, despite the fact that girls attend college at much higher rates than boys (Buchmann, DiPrete, & McDaniel, 2008). The gendered nature of the full Disruption of Difference model likely arose because girls, as a group, are better students and harder to get off the college track. On the other hand, boys face more difficulty in high school and are much more likely to be derailed on the track to college. Thus, for girls, the social and emotional difficulties of high school may be the only thing powerful enough to hurt them. For boys, however, these difficulties are merely a drop in the bucket of things that threaten their futures.

Locating Mechanisms

What I have discussed so far suggests that stigma raises the risk of the full Disruption of Difference pathway for girls and part of the Disruption of Difference pathway for boys. Yet, both girls and boys vary in how they react to social stigma. That variability is important because knowing who gets disrupted, and why, helps us figure out developmentally informed plans of action in schools. To delve into this variability, consider what the intervening steps in that link between social stigma and short-term coping mechanisms might be. In particular, how is stigma activated in schools, why does such activation matter, and when does it not matter? These questions touch on highly personal, quite nuanced issues that are difficult to capture in the kinds of surveys employed by national studies such as Add Health. Consequently, the adolescents at Lamar offer the best means for answering these questions. Through interviews, creative projects (e.g., making Who I Am collages), and guided tours through social networking sites, they revealed many important insights into the issues at hand.

Beginning with the issue of how messages of difference are transmitted to adolescents, adolescents' own attempts at social comparison were important. What appeared to be the strongest *peer* vectors of transmission of these messages, however, was the feedback that they received on two general levels of high school social life.

First, even though many socially marginalized youth have no friends, some do, and those friendship dynamics can be tricky. Reflecting a common tendency among American adolescents (Giordano, 2003), the students at Lamar idealized their friendship groups and made claims that, to quote one young Latina, their friends "accept me for who I am" and "do not try to change me." Nevertheless, most adolescents, when pressed, acknowledged that their friends had ways of policing them, of letting them know when they may have been at risk of social troubles at school.

This policing, however, had a positive spin to it, in the form of joking or offers to help. Thus, friends could give negative messages camouflaged by warm feelings.

Second, Lamar youth could also map out the larger bands of peer crowds and status groups that cut across the student body. These bands of peers, which encompassed many different cliques and served as pools of potential friends and romantic partners to anyone in their orbit, were almost universally viewed by adolescents at Lamar as the level of the peer world in which social exclusion and the punishment of difference happened. This viewpoint reflects the basic insights of work by psychologists and sociologists (Barber et al., 2001; Frank et al., 2008) that adolescents are more at risk in diffuse peer groupings than among friends because, absent strong emotional ties that characterize the former, they are more expendable for breaking norms. The Lamar adolescents came to a rough consensus on the means by which these larger bands of peers regulated conformity and nonconformity in the school – private talk directed outward, double speak, third-person comments, dirty looks – and overwhelmingly recognized that girls were much better at the carrying out these means than boys. Importantly, they also agreed that such subtle or at least plausibly denial acts of aggression and exclusion were far more effective at policing difference than overt acts of hostility or harassment. As one young woman explained, sometimes she thought something was happening but could never be sure, and that uncertainty and nagging doubt seemed far worse to her than actually knowing what others thought of her.

Turning to the issue of why messages of difference matter, the Lamar adolescents helped explain that negative social feedback from peers triggered problematic coping responses by complicating how they viewed themselves. Reflecting the basic principles of classic social psychological theories of the self (Baumeister, 1998), the adolescents at Lamar were constantly trying to integrate all of the complex and occasionally contradictory information coming at them from different directions into a cohesive picture of identity. They also recognized that their time at Lamar and who they met there played a major role in this process. Although all of the adolescents had undergone some struggles, the ones who were the most troubled were those who felt as though they were boiled down into a single characteristic, especially a devalued one like being overweight or economically disadvantaged, by others at school, that they were judged according to a simplistic label. These feelings illustrate Goffman's (1963) notion of spoiled identity or more recent conceptualizations of identity discrepancy (Ewell, Smith, Karmel, & Hart, 1996). These disruptions in identity development, in turn, require work – identity work – to fix, such as through internalization (an attempt to promote consistency between self and social perceptions at any cost), self-medication (an attempt to neutralize discrepancies between self and social perceptions), and disengagement (an attempt to shield self perceptions from social perceptions). This identity work, in turn, competes with school work.

Finally, as for situations in which messages of difference will not matter, the adolescents at Lamar came up with an exhaustive list of personal, social, and institutional resources that they thought would enable an adolescent to cope in the short term with social problems at high school in ways that did not create long-term consequences. As best as the data allowed, I tested their hypotheses about resources for resilience with Add Health, attempting to identify factors that reduced the problematic links between obesity and poverty on the one hand and aspects of internalization, self-medication, and disengagement on the other. School activity participation (including sports) and other kinds of out-of-school activities/hobbies (again including sports) appeared to provide a protective function for both girls and boys, as did having close friends and romantic partners. What I found for various kinds of family resources was more complex. Although having supportive, involved parents and cohesive families was associated with better socioe-motional functioning for adolescents in general, this family resource had less of an observed effect on obese and/or poor youth than on other youth. Thus, both the at-risk and non-at-risk groups did better when exposed to this family resource, but, because this improvement was greater for the latter than the former, the gap between the at-risk and non-at-risk groups actually widened. In sum, the main "trigger" in the Disruption of Difference was not inevitable, suggesting that, for some adolescents and in some high schools, the link between problems on the social side of school and their academic prospects was not unbreakable.

CONCLUSION

The full pattern of Disruption of Difference among girls and the partial pattern among boys reflects the fact that adolescents, like adults, are highly social actors with strong agentic impulses but often short-sighted perspectives on life. As such, they actively evaluate themselves in a social arena that can create positive/negative psychological states that then need to be maintained or treated in ways that produce different consequences depending on the short term versus the long term. Although we can view this phenomenon as somewhat timeless in many ways, we can also think about how the contours of this game have changed. First, in the impersonal nature of the modern high school and the expansion of high school peer culture onto a virtual plane, short-cut tricks to categorize and evaluate people take on added value and make spoiled identities more likely. Second, in a changed educational and economic landscape, the distractions that these sort of struggles have always caused can now prove to be near-fatal academic blows. Thus, we have a personal process of psychosocial development that plays out in the proximate settings of ecology (e.g., peer groups, schools), but this "playing out" is shaped by larger structure of society and, in the aggregate, contributes to the form and function of this structure. This two-way, bottom-down/top-up influence captures the sociological concept of structuration and is akin to Piaget's concept of equilibrium.

Understanding this process helps us understand development in an abstract, theoretical sense but also helps us take a more developmentally grounded approach to policy. For example, the Disruption of Difference suggests the potential value of school size reductions, expanded extracurricula, and on-site mental health services. As another example, it also suggests the folly of pushing academic reforms and behavioral interventions without sufficient recognition of the social context of the schools in which they will be enacted. In other words, educational policy will benefit and our service of adolescents will be improved when the view of high school in the United States is expanded, in a practical sense, from training/credentialing institution to developmental context.

Beyond theory and policy, we can also use insights about the role of high schools as developmental contexts in the modern era as a way of grounding our perceptions of young people and their lives in their own realities. This is useful for adults who, upon hearing an adolescent complain about the pressures of adolescent society, are prone to think that this is merely a rite of passage. It is also useful for adults who, upon reading rankings of the "best" high schools in the United States, such as the annual report by *Newsweek*, might forget that school quality is defined by more than standardized test passing rates and Advanced Placement course offerings.

ACKNOWLEDGMENTS

The author acknowledges the generous support of a faculty scholar award from the William T. Grant Foundation and grants from the National Institute of Child Health and Human Development (R03 HD047378–01, PI: Robert Crosnoe; R24 HD042849, PI: Mark Hayward).

REFERENCES

Adler, P. & Adler, P. (1998). *Peer power: Preadolescent culture and identity.* New Brunswick, NJ: Rutgers.

Akerlof, G. E. & Kranton, R. A. (2002). Identity and schooling: Some lessons for the economics of education. *Journal of Economic Literature, 40,* 1167–1201.

Allen, J. P., Porter, M. R., McFarland, C. F., Marsh, P., & McElhaney, K. B. (2005). The two faces of adolescents' success with peers: Adolescent popularity, social adaptation, and deviant behavior. *Child Development, 76,* 747–760.

Attewell, P. & Domina, T. (2008). Raising the bar: Curricular intensity and academic performance. *Educational Evaluation and Policy Analysis, 30,* 51–71.

Bandura, A. (2001). Social cognitive theory: An agentic perspective. *Annual Review of Psychology, 52,* 1–26.

Barber, B. L., Eccles, J. S., & Stone, M. R. (2001). Whatever happened to the jock, the brain, and the princess?: Young adult pathways linked to adolescent activity involvement and social identity. *Journal of Adolescent Research, 16,* 429–455.

Baum, S. & Ma, J. (2007). *Education pays: The benefits of higher education for individuals and society.* Washington, DC: College Board.

Baumeister, R. (1998). The self. In J. Howard & P. Callero (Eds.), *Handbook of social psychology* (4th Ed., pp. 680–740). Cambridge: Cambridge University Press.

Bearman, P. S. & Bruckner, H. (2001). Promising the future: Virginity pledges and first intercourse. *American Journal of Sociology, 106,* 859–912.

Bernhardt, A., Morris, M., Handcock, M. S., & Scott, M. A. (2001). *Divergent paths: Economic mobility in the new American labor market.* New York: Russell Sage.

Brown, B., Green, N., & Harper, R. (Eds.). (2002). *Wireless world: Social and interactional aspects of the mobile age.* London: Springer.

Brown, B. B. & Klute, C. (2003). Friendships, cliques, and crowds. In G. Adams & M. D. Berzonsky (Eds.), *Blackwell handbook of adolescence* (pp. 330–348). Malden, MA: Blackwell.

Brumberg, J. J. (1997). *The body project: An intimate history of American girls.* New York: Random House.

Buchmann, B., DiPrete, T. A., & McDaniel, A. (2008). Gender inequalities in education. *Annual Review of Sociology, 34,* 319–337.

Carter, P. (2006). *Keepin' it real: School success beyond black and white.* New York: Oxford University Press.

Centers for Disease Control and Prevention. (2000). Body mass index. Online at http://www.cdc.gov/nccdphp/dnpa/bmi

Coleman, J. (1961). *The adolescent society.* New York: Free Press of Glencoe.

Crandall, C. (1994). Prejudice against fat people: Ideology and self-interest. *Journal of Personality and Social Psychology, 66,* 882–894.

Crosnoe, R. (2006). The connection between academic failure and adolescent drinking in secondary school. *Sociology of Education, 79,* 44–60.

(2011). *Fitting in, standing out: Navigating the social challenges of high school to get an education.* New York: Cambridge University Press.

Crosnoe, R., Muller, C., & Frank, K. (2004). Peer context and the consequences of adolescent drinking. *Social Problems, 51,* 288–304.

Dance, T. L. (2002). *Tough fronts: The impact of street culture on schooling.* New York: Routledge.

Darling-Hammond, L. (2006). No Child Left Behind and high school reform. *Harvard Educational Review, 76*(4), 642–667.

Duncan, G. J., Brooks-Gunn, J., Yeung, W. J., & Smith, J. R. (1998). How much does childhood poverty affect the life chances of children? *American Sociological Review, 63*, 406–423.

Eccles, J. & Barber, B. (1999). Student council, volunteering, basketball, or marching band: What kind of extracurricular involvement matters? *Journal of Adolescent Research, 14*, 10–43.

Eccles, J. S. & Wigfield, A. (2002). Motivational beliefs, values, and goals. *Annual Review of Psychology, 53*, 109–132.

Eckert, P. (1989). *Jocks and burnouts: Social identity in the high school.* New York: Teachers College Press.

Eder, D., Evans, C., & Parker, S. (1995). *School talk: Gender and adolescent culture.* New Brunswick, NJ: Rutgers.

Elder, G. H. (1998). The life course as developmental theory. *Child Development, 69*, 1–12.

Ewell, F., Smith, S., Karmel, M. P., & Hart, D. (1996). The sense of self and its development: A framework for understanding eating disorders. In L. Smolak, M. P. Levine, & R. Striegel-Moor (Eds.), *The developmental psychopathology of eating disorders: Implications for research, prevention, and treatment* (pp. 107–133). Mahwah, NJ: Erlbaum.

Fischer, C. S. & Hout, M. (2006). *Century of difference: How America changed in the last one hundred years.* New York: Russell Sage.

Frank, K. A., Muller, C., Schiller, K. S., Riegle-Crumb, C., Mueller, A. S., Crosnoe, R., & Pearson, J. (2008). The social dynamics of mathematics coursetaking in high school. *American Journal of Sociology, 113*, 1645–1696.

Furstenberg, F. F. (2000). The sociology of adolescence and youth in the 1990s: A critical commentary. *Journal of Marriage and Family, 62*, 896–910.

Giordano, P. C. (2003). Relationships in adolescence. *Annual Review of Sociology, 29*, 257–281.

Goffman, E. (1963). *Stigma: Notes on the management of spoiled identity.* Englewood Cliffs, NJ: Prentice-Hall.

Goldin, C. & Katz, L. F. (2008). *The race between technology and education.* Cambridge, MA: Harvard University Press.

Goldsmith, P. A. (2004). Schools' racial mix, students' optimism, and the black-white and latino-white achievement gaps. *Sociology of Education, 77*, 121–147.

Greenfield, P. & Yan, Z. (2006). Children, adolescents, and the internet: A new field of inquiry in developmental psychology. *Developmental Psychology, 3*, 391–394.

Guyer, A. E., McClure-Tone, E. B., Shiffrin, N. D., Pine, D. S., Nelson, E. E. (2009). Probing the neural correlates of anticipated peer evaluation in adolescence. *Child Development, 80*, 1000–1015.

Harris, K. M. (2008). *The National Longitudinal Study of Adolescent Health, Waves I & II, 1994–1996; Wave III, 2001–2002.* Chapel Hill, NC: Carolina Population Center, University of North Carolina at Chapel Hill.

Hegerty, P. (2009). Toward an LGBT-informed paradigm of children who break gender norms. *Developmental Psychology, 45,* 895–900.

Hernandez, D., Denton, N., & Macartney, S. (2007). Children in immigrant families. *SRCD Social Policy Report, 22,* 3–22.

Hussong, A. M., Hicks, R. E., Levy, S. A., & Curran, P. J. (2001). Specifying the relations between affect and heavy alcohol use among young adults. *Journal of Abnormal Psychology, 110,* 449–461.

Johnson, M. K., Crosnoe, R., & Elder, Jr., G. H. (2001). Students' attachment and academic engagement: The role of ethnicity. *Sociology of Education, 74,* 318–340.

Kinney, D. (1999). From "headbangers" to "hippies": Delineating adolescents' active attempts to form an alternative peer culture. *New Directions for Child and Adolescent Development, 84,* 21–35.

Kraut, R. E., Patterson, M., Lundmark, V., Kiesler, S., Mukhopadhyay, T., & Scherlis, W. (1998). Internet paradox: A social technology that reduces social involvement and psychological well-being? *American Psychologist, 53*(9), 1017–1032.

La Greca, A. M. & Lopez, N. (1998). Social anxiety among adolescents: Linkages with peer relations and friendships. *Journal of Abnormal Child Psychology, 26,* 83–94.

Labaree, D. F. (1997). Public goods, private goods: The American struggle over educational goals. *American Educational Research Journal, 34,* 39–81.

Lee, V., Smith, J., & Croninger, R. (1997). How high school organization influences the equitable distribution of learning in mathematics and science. *Sociology of Education, 70,* 128–150.

Lenhart, A. (2008). Teens and media use: An overview. Pew Internet and American Life Project. Online at http://www.pewinternet.org/Presentations/2009/17-Teens-and-Social-Media-An-Overview.aspx

Lightfoot, S. L. (1983). *The good high school: Portraits of character and culture.* New York: Basic Books.

Link, B. G. & Phelan, J. C. (2001). Conceptualizing stigma. *Annual Review of Sociology, 27,* 363–385.

McFarland, D. A. & Pals, H. (2005). Motives and contexts of identity change: A case for network effects. *Social Psychology Quarterly, 68,* 289–315.

McLanahan, S. (2004). Children and the second demographic transition. *Demography, 41,* 607–628.

McLoyd, V. C. (1998). Socioeconomic disadvantage and child development. *American Psychologist, 53,* 185–204.

McNeely, C., Nonnemaker, J., & Blum, R. (2002). Promoting student connectedness to school: Evidence from the National Longitudinal Study of Adolescent Health. *Journal of School Health, 72,* 138–146.

Milner, M. (2004). *Freaks, geeks, and cool kids: American teenagers, schools, and the culture of consumption.* New York: Routledge.

Mirowsky, J. & Ross, C. E. (2003). *Social causes of psychological distress: Second edition.* New York: Aldine de Gruyter.

Modell, J. (1989). *Into one's own: From youth to adulthood in the United States, 1920–1975.* Berkeley: University of California Press.

Morgan, S. L. 2005. *On the Edge of Commitment: Educational Attainment and Race in the United States.* Stanford, CA: Stanford University Press.

National Academy of Sciences. (2007). *Rising above the gathering storm. Energizing and employing America for a brighter future.* Washington, DC: National Academies Press.

Powell, A. G., Farrar, E., & Cohen, D. K. (1985). *The shopping mall high school: Winners and losers in the educational marketplace.* Boston, MA: Houghton-Mifflin.

Puhl, R. & Brownell, K. D. (2001). Bias, discrimination, and obesity. *Obesity Research, 9,* 788–805.

Roeser, R. & Eccles, J. S. (2000). Schooling and mental health. In A. J. Sameroff, M. Lewis, & S. Miller (Eds.), *Handbook of developmental psychopathology* (pp. 135–156). Dordrecht: Kluwer.

Ross, C. E. (1994). Overweight and depression. *Journal of Health and Social Behavior, 33,* 63–78.

Rudolph, K. D. & Conley, C. S. (2005). The socioemotional costs and benefits of social-evaluative concerns: Do girls care too much? *Journal of Personality, 73,* 115–138.

Sandstrom, M. J., Cillessen, A. H., & Eisenhower, A. (2003). Children's appraisal of peer rejection experiences: Impact on social and emotional adjustment. *Social Development, 12,* 530–550.

Schneider, B. (2007). *Forming a college-going community in U.S. schools.* Seattle, WA: Bill and Melinda Gates Foundation.

Steinberg, L. D. (2001). We know some things: Parent-adolescent relationships in retrospect and prospect. *Journal of Research on Adolescence, 11,* 1–20.

(2008). A social neuroscience perspective on adolescent risk-taking. *Developmental Review, 28,* 78–106.

Steinberg, L. D., Brown, B. B., & Dornbusch, S. M. (1996). *Beyond the classroom: Why school reform has failed and what parents need to do.* New York: Simon & Schuster.

Suzuki, L. K. & Calzo, J. P. (2004). The search for peer advice in cyberspace: An examination of online teen bulletin boards about health and sexuality. *Journal of Applied Developmental Psychology, 25,* 685–698.

U.S. Census Bureau. (2007). Current Population Survey reports: School enrollment. Online at http://www.census.gov/population/www/socdemo/school.html

U.S. Census Bureau. (2009). Poverty: Definitions. Online at http://www.census.gov/hhes/www/poverty/definitions.html

Weinstein, R. (2002). *Reaching higher: The power of expectations in schooling.* Cambridge, MA: Harvard University Press.

Yeung, K. T. & Martin, J. L. (2003). The looking glass self: An empirical test and elaboration. *Social Forces, 81,* 843–879.

Zhou, M. (1997). Growing up American: The challenge confronting immigrant children and children of immigrants. *Annual Review of Sociology, 23,* 63–95.

Index

**Published by Lawrence Erlbaum Associates/ Taylor
and Francis/ Psychology Press** (*continued from page iii*)

Conceptual Development: Piaget's Legacy, edited by Ellin Kofsky Scholnick, Katherine Nelson, Susan A. Gelman, and Patricia H. Miller, 1999.

Change and Development: Issues of Theory, Method, and Application, edited by Eric Amsel and K. Ann Renninger, 1997.

Piaget, Evolution, and Development, edited by Jonas Langer and Melanie Killen, 1998.

Values and Knowledge, edited by Edward S. Reed, Elliot Turiel, and Terrance Brown, 1996.

Development and Vulnerability in Close Relationships, edited by Gil G. Noam and Kurt W. Fischer, 1996.

The Nature and Ontogenesis of Meaning, edited by Willis F. Overton and David S. Palermo, 1994.

Development in Context: Acting and Thinking in Specific Environments, edited by Robert H. Wozniak and Kurt W. Fischer, 1993.

Piaget's Theory: Prospects and Possibilities, edited by Harry Beilin and Peter B. Pufall, 1992.

The Epigenesis of Mind: Essays on Biology and Cognition, edited by Susan Carey and Rochel Gelman, 1991.

Constructivist Perspectives on Developmental Psychopathology and Atypical Development, edited by Daniel P. Keating and Hugh Rosen, 1990.

Reasoning, Necessity, and Logic: Developmental Perspectives, edited by Willis F. Overton, 1990.

Constructivism in the Computer Age, edited by George Forman and Peter B. Pufall, 1988.

Development and Learning: Conflict or Congruence? edited by Lynn S. Liben, 1987.

Thought and Emotion: Developmental Perspectives, edited by D. J. Bearison and H. Zimiles, 1985.

Moderators of Competence, edited by Edith D. Neimark, R. De Lisi, and Judith L. Newman, 1985.

New Trends in Conceptual Representation: Challenges to Piaget's Theory? edited by Ellin Kofsky Scholnick, 1983.

Piaget and the Foundations of Knowledge, edited by Lynn S. Liben, 1983.

The Relationship Between Social and Cognitive Development, edited by Willis F. Overton, 1983.

New Directions in Piagetian Theory and Practice, edited by Irving E. Sigel, David M. Brodzinsky, and Roberta M. Golinkoff, 1981.